Less Than Human

James Gannon MD

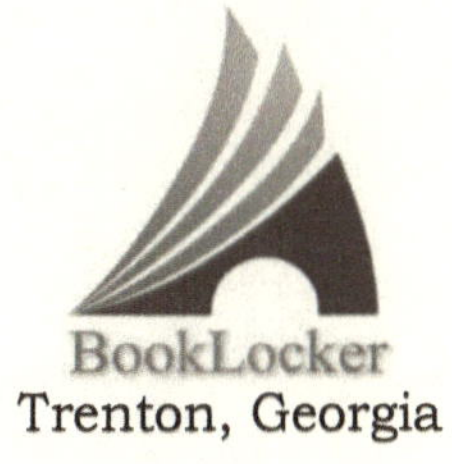

BookLocker
Trenton, Georgia

Print ISBN: 978-1-958889-02-2
Ebook ISBN: 979-8-88531-451-0

Published by BookLocker.com, Inc., Trenton, Georgia, U.S.A.

Printed on acid-free paper.

Library of Congress Cataloguing in Publication Data
Gannon MD, James
Less Than Human by James Gannon MD
Library of Congress Control Number: 2023901625

BookLocker.com, Inc.
2023

Second Edition

Dedication

To Angela, my wife: Too many years were spent apart
during medical training. I miss every one of those days
away from your loving arms and smiling face. Thanks for
being you.

To the others fighting to provide humane
compassionate patient care in this dehumanizing
era, of fast protocol medicine, thank you.

In loving memory of an influential high school teacher,
Ned Livengood: he stimulated thought in young students
by frequently asking, "what is the significance?" I hope
you, the reader find some significance in this work.

Contents

Less than Human

Prologue

Much of the examples contained in this book focus on experiences and analysis prior to the first edition release in 2015 and most of that content remains relevant today.

This story is based on experience. With the exception of references from public domain the names are excluded to protect anyone from personal harm.

I do not claim to be perfect or that mine is the only side of the story. I stand before you a sample of human imperfection, but still try to leave the world just a little bit of a better place than I found it. It is common to belittle those who complain about abusive systems and decry those persons as weak and failures. I am a success within the system, yet can describe serious, unaddressed issues in the education, healthcare, media and political systems, which essentially encompasses any hierarchy that extols absolute responsibility on persons who have no actual authority and allows those in positions of power to avoid accountability. Those observations were true with my original edition and remain true today. My efforts as a physician help lives on an individual level but I hope this document makes people think and initiate positive changes on a systemic level in our healthcare, education and political-media systems beyond the agenda-driven propaganda existing today. I wish this could be a story about amusing medical anecdotes, but medical practice has been so overwhelmed by economic, media, political and legal factors that no mention of medicine can be made without reference to such factors and how they impact the healthcare field.

Part 1:

Getting There

Chapter 1
A Calling

Everyone has some calling of benefit to the world, and one needs to pursue that calling. I have found the hard way that holding one's self back from trying is worse than any failed attempt at accomplishment. For example, if one fails to become an engineer due to not being able to handle the profession's mathematic rigors, one still at least has exposure to higher math and a better respect for the profession. Also, the alternate degree pathways for those who drop out of engineering still can be quite lucrative. One teacher called it "the sieve of engineering and the trampoline of accounting." Point was, many engineering "drop-outs" still have something to break their fall, and they do well in life. In contrast, if one decides not to advance academically or attempt some other life venture for fear of failure, then those opportunities are lost.

The proper amount of fear can prevent you from doing something stupid and potentially dangerous, but too much fear can be self-destructive.

Finally, I recall a chemistry book in which each chapter had a brief page of successful people relating a chemistry story. More than one of those stories mentioned how Organic Chemistry ("O-Chem" in school jargon) was the stumbling block leading to a change in degree major. If memory serves correct, one became a very successful biologist, another became a very successful computer artist modeling science topics, and a third became a technical writer. Hence, these are people who have adapted to an educationally adverse situation and still became quite successful. My point is this: Failure is guaranteed if you do not try- you must try.

At some point in life, a calling grabs you. Sometimes it is how you picture yourself in the world, other times it is a nagging restlessness that indicates you are not in a position to just stop and feel self-fulfilled. What are your innate talents and are you using them? How do you define your contribution in society and how do you become that definition? Not all roads lead to your goals, and along the way are many diversions, pitfalls and fears. Attending college and professional school in the United States is huge money and even with achieving a successful degree, the venture can carry a crippling cost. Of course, the bone-crushing student loan debt hurts a bit worse when certain politicians want to use your tax dollars to give criminals a free college education, which is what you leveraged your entire financial future upon. When you are done with college, there is no guarantee of a certain job or social status, which makes you wonder if you did the right thing.

Yet, investing in yourself is always the right thing, because what you are is the only thing some thief or government bureau cannot take away from you. Try to meld your skills and knowledge with your inherent talent. Sometimes fear of failure is paralyzing, but it must be overcome. You may not have things work out as planned, but something will work out; put your faith in God, not man. If you think of your formal and informal education as developing and honing your personal human skill set, you will be prepared to adapt and improvise to changing situations better than if you are just looking for one specific role out of your training. I once saw a motivational plaque on a wall stating, *Luck is where preparation meets opportunity.* You cannot guarantee luck, but you can "be prepared."

Chapter 2
Higher Education

Unfortunately, much of the education system is more of an antagonistic challenge than a training process. Some assignments and exams appear designed deliberately tough so that everyone fails and only the good will of the professor, via the class bell curve, rescues you from disaster. Such an academic system seems harmful, because you never feel you really learned anything; you just feel you got through it. Also, rather than developing collegiality in mastering the material, often each student is pitted against the others. The education process is more like martial arts sparring training than a teaching process; perhaps one should co
nsider higher education sort of a mental sparring match.

You must learn to teach yourself, to be an initiator, not a sponge. I have observed that a young mind does absorb information much like a sponge but often does not grasp the significance of the information. As we age, we more fully synthesize information and grasp the meaning, but do not as readily absorb such quantities of information as when we were young. Such a situation indicates inherent ways in which the brain functions and implies proper utilization of those abilities at the ideal time can optimize the learning process.

Yet, the academic system often skips the process of teaching you how to become a self-learner and hopes such abilities will magically come to you one day. I had a philosophy teacher state, "I cannot teach you how to think, but I can teach you to think." At another time, a physics instructor stated, "I cannot teach you to think, but I can teach you how to think." Hence, the right combination of art and science, abstract reasoning, and concrete calculations of physical relationships seems to be able to bridge the gap between teaching someone to think and teaching them how to think.

Primary education could perhaps better utilize the brain developmental timing discordance between concrete and abstract learning to maximize the ability of young people to memorize many languages and facts and a bit later use those known facts of knowledge in teaching abstract math concepts. For example, arbitrary learning of physics waveforms and nuances of light diffraction means nothing to a lot of people, and is not necessary for learning music and art. Yet, at some point, teaching waveform physics in the context of musical string instruments and optics as related to photography, art and vision may increase the appreciation of both art and science and add interesting concrete examples to formerly abstract ideas.

Regardless whether your education is a nurturing or challenging process, you must press on, for you have a calling.

For a few students, the pressure of higher education becomes too much and they kill themselves. As one person stated to me, "Suicide is a permanent answer to a temporary problem." You do not need perfection for success. For example, I had a situation where I was doing well in a class and the final exam was the day before Thanksgiving. When you work in a grocery store, getting the day before Thanksgiving off would require divine intervention, which did not happen. As I was about to ask the teacher if the final exam could be taken at a different time, another student beat me to the same question. Yes, it was an example of a teacher being antagonistic to students who actually worked their way through college. The professor's answer was that "no exceptions" were to be made, and the time stated was the only time to take the final exam, period. I could not take the final exam. By my calculations, even if I got a zero on the final exam, the calculated grade result would be at least a D and most likely a low C, because I had good grades going into the final exam. The unexpected happened. Not being able to take the final exam, I received a grade of "Incomplete" for the entire quarter of class. Yes, attending every lecture and having A's or high B's on all but one exam is Incomplete by academic standards. I later became aware that by school policy all "Incomplete" grades eventually became an F.

Another time, I signed up for a class that was a basic electric circuits course, which was redundant given classes I had before in trade school, but the junior college would not accept my trade school circuits courses as meeting the requirement for a certain associate degree track I was considering. The class affected my work schedule to a great extent. The class became ridiculous, because the teacher would get tied up with one pair of students on one simple question and most of a 4-5 hour Saturday morning class was spent just waiting for the instructor to turn on the power switch or unlock the cabinet to get a battery to run the circuit we assembled. Since the quarter began on Monday and the last day to get a full refund was Friday, it was a past the refundable drop date by the first day of class. I ceased attending after two wasted Saturdays. Since there was no refund, I did not try to take unpaid time off work to go through the official drop process. Failure to officially drop a course resulted in an Incomplete, which then became an F. Those F's hit the GPA calculations hard, but I still had a respectable GPA. Of course, I later became much more cautious regarding the nuances of academic bureaucracy in regards to grading schemes.

Those F's also hit hard decades later while applying to medical school, because at one school someone actually asked me about it. I was a bit shocked that a couple F's from junior college around 1982 and 1983 would be an issue in 1998-99 interview season, since even with those 2 F's I still had earned two associate degrees with well above 3.0 GPA while working full-time and was currently a full-time cum laude student in an esteemed engineering program at a well-regarded school. The academic system can be punitive and unforgiving but my dream was not destroyed.

Point is, if I can overcome two F's and still get into professional school, so can you. Please, do not kill yourself over a school grade, because it is not worth it. You are more than an academic number.

The most desirable colleges are competitive, and an academic pedigree has its privileges, but all education is useful. As one guy said to me, "What do they call the lowest ranked graduate in the least regarded medical school? The answer is 'Doctor.'" The point is once you are out practicing your career, you will be evaluated in most part by your personal performance, not your academic pedigree. Hence, although academic pedigree can help open some doors, it is not the only factor in success. Also, academic pedigree can be obtained anywhere along the way, be it undergraduate education, professional school training, residency programs, research programs, certificate programs and even honorary degrees. Thus, do not be crushed if you do not get your most desired program; there is always a side door, back door, window or another day.

Not all school is studying, there is some fun, but there is also plenty of distraction, injustice and tragedy to go around. After all, real life things such as lying, cheating, stealing, racial slurs, suicide and even rape happen in the best of places.

The hardest compromise of having been a working adult and subsequently going back into the education system full-time was the complete forfeiture of civil rights. You should not have to compromise your civil rights in the U.S. to obtain college education. In fact, as Americans we are, or at least we were, conditioned to never compromise on your civil rights, unfortunately things have changed since my high school American Government/Civics class in the late 1970's. Apparently each professor is given god-like status over his or her academic sphere of influence and as a student you have no right to contest. I had issues with one godhead professor, but complaints to the dean were fruitless. In my situation, I had taken an interesting graduate-level class while an undergraduate student. Many of the professor's own graduate students were in the class, and the overt preference he gave them was occasionally sickening. Some of them could not speak comprehensible English and often rambled close to an hour on a "20-minute presentation" yet were praised greatly by this obviously-biased professor. Some of his graduate students read their presentation verbatim from a paper they copied and placed on the overhead projector and if asked a question, went directly back to iterating the sentence or paragraph verbatim and never actually answered the question. Never mind the paper they were reading was directly from an article the presenter never properly cited or was evidently completely done by someone else because the person doing the presentation seemed to have no clue as to what they were reciting. Yes, many of those people likely have become U.S. college professors and are probably the ones American students complain they cannot understand. The person(s) complaining about the incomprehensible professor often end up labeled a bigot or racist for expecting U.S. college professors to be able to communicate to American students. I realize that desiring teachers in the United States to actually speak comprehensibly in English now makes me a bigot, a hater, and many other insults hurled at people who point out the ludicrousness of the situation. Small wonder the United States has such a difficult time educating its youth – no one can understand half of what many of the professors are saying. Education requires communication, and if the professor cannot speak the language, an interpreter should be provided.

The last straw in that class was regarding a term paper, which was a considerable portion of the class grade. I tried several times to contact the professor for input to my document preparation, all to no avail. I emailed him the document, but he did not look at it. Attempted to schedule an appointment, but he had no time. I tried to talk after class, but again no time for me. I gave him a printed hard copy to review at his discretion, yet again no feedback from the professor. To me, it seems very discriminatory to isolate a single student or student population in your class and refuse to advise him or them, while at the same time overtly providing all sorts of access to another student population. So, I did the entire term paper without any input from the professor. In the end, he gave me a relatively average grade for what I thought was exceptional work. The term paper result lowered my overall class grade considerably, and the only comments he made on the term paper was, "too many quotes." He evidently had no other negative comments about the term paper, because "too many quotes" was the only markings on the entire document.

I complained about the plagiarism, extra time for his students on presentations and the fact that the professor refused my many attempts by several methods to communicate in preparation for my term paper, then seemed to take off an inordinate amount of grading for using "too many quotes." My complaints fell on deaf ears, as the dean informed me, "The professors can run their classes anyway they like." Afterwards, I had written a rather scathing email and in one part indicated the school should be ashamed as it had perpetually driven a student to suicide almost every semester, but that one day the school administration would cause someone to go the other way (implying, not suicide, but homicide). History has too often proven me correct, not just at my school, but at too many schools.

As an example of how few rights a student has, I offer this story. I saw a graduate student, who mentored one of our lab sessions, walking across the campus on a summer day. I said "hello" but then noticed he seemed infuriated. He informed me his professor came in that morning and stated, "Why do I have you here, I don't need you anymore." Just like that, several years of Ph.D. research efforts taken away, his career ended. He already had a Master's degree and was working toward a Ph.D. A fact that made the sting even worse was that during a previous conversation this graduate student mentioned to me he was lured away from a different department to work with this professor – yes, this guy who just fired him. When he saw me, he was walking to an administrative office to apply for a "Plan B" Master's degree, his second Master's degree. He did not go on a violent killing spree, but one Ph.D. candidate, Wlodzimierz Dedecjus, did kill his professor in 1998 for allegedly blocking Mr. Wlodzimierz's graduation. In 1978, Ted Streleski was 19 years into his mathematics doctorate and killed a professor, considering his actions a political statement regarding the poor treatment of graduate students.

A few years after I had graduated, a terrible situation occurred at my former college. A person somehow chronically related to the university claimed his computer website was being maliciously hacked into with derogatory ethnic and religious insults. This was before such activity was formally classified as a hate crime. This self-proclaimed victim of a computer hacking made his accusations and felt the school did nothing to address the issue and may have even considered the school officials covered for the alleged perpetrator (It would not surprise me if his assumptions were entirely correct.). He is reported to have subsequently sued the school for an enormous amount. Based on the ludicrous amount of the damages claimed in the lawsuit, the judge threw the case out of court. I later read an online blog stating that man even wrote a personal note to the judge requesting that the case be reinstated or the insulted party would have to take matters into his own hands. On May 9, 2003, Mr. Biswanath Holder did flip out, for lack of a better description, and took a gun into a building and started shooting. An innocent person was killed and two others were injured. I do not know if the man had a history of mental illness, but I do know that school administration can push people to the limits and that can end in tragedy, usually with totally innocent persons becoming the victims. Since that time, we have had plenty more examples of such violence, yet at no time have the school officials been called to task for the hostile environment they create, which fosters such tragedies and abuses.

For a racism incident brushed under the rug by school administrators, I offer Monkeys and Squirrels. A black student was running for student council, and in many places he and his supporters posted his name in chalk (aka "chalking," where temporary student notices/announcements are written on sidewalks and sides of objects in chalk). All the other candidates had their names in chalk, too. Well, some of the black guy's chalkings had his name crossed out and the word "monkey" written next to his name. This incident was in the late 1990s in Ohio at a renowned university, not stereotypical pre-1960s Ku Klux Klan territory. Obviously, it was improper behavior and could certainly be construed as racially-motivated, racially- insensitive, potentially racially-hostile, and even overt racism. When the offenders of some fraternity were caught, they offered up the explanation that they were simply playing a game called "Monkeys and Squirrels" – except, there were no squirrels. No other people's names had their name crossed out and the word "squirrel" or "monkey" placed next to it. Well, that was good enough for school administration, no racism here, just a little misunderstanding. We, the students did subsequently have a meeting about racism, which for some students was more revealing regarding administrative lying. The university president was not at this meeting, and when other administrators were questioned if the president did not think a meeting about racism was important enough to attend, the ensuing defense of the president's absence was absolutely refuted by physical facts pointed out by one very astute graduate student and a hush fell over the crowd, except for whispers of young students in front of me stating, "Oh my God, he's lying." When a perception of justice, of right and wrong, is so warped and no one in power does the right thing, people lose faith and feel the need to take matters into their own hands; as indicated before, the unaddressed injustice can often turn tragic under vigilante justice. None of these atrocities surprise me in a situation where students and other underlings have no civil rights and administrators and professors are like unaccountable gods and demigods.

As a student, all you can do is realize you are powerless to change the academic juggernaut, and so you continue on your pathway. Sure, you may need to speak up for what is right and condemn what is wrong, knowing full well your integrity will be used against you. The best thing I can advise is to make your complaints in writing through proper channels; it may not accomplish anything in your academic lifetime but may help others later, and it will leave a record that something was in fact said, so the administrators cannot hide under the veil of feigned ignorance, as is most often the case.

Not everyone has bad experiences, and almost no one has all bad experiences, but you may as well know at least a small bit of the truth about higher education. Regardless, keep focused on your dreams, goals and callings, and adjust as necessary. I did not say it was easy, but you can succeed.

Chapter 3
Roadblocks and Extortion

Let us face it, a lot of college curriculum is game playing to make more money and to act as roadblocks for applicants applying to professional programs. The roadblocks to other fields of endeavor actually made achieving my goal of becoming a doctor easier and more focused. For example, the prerequisites for fields like pharmacy and physician assistant were quite inconsistent. Every pharmacy and physician assistant program in the country seemed to each have at least a few different requirements, which were usually not even related to the final degree. Medicine was actually easier and more standardized regarding fulfilling pre-requisites. Medical schools wanted you to have some basic biology, general chemistry, one to two semesters of organic chemistry, organic chemistry laboratory, one year of physics at any level, and math up to at least one calculus course. No medical school candidate was denied because the person did not take a course like "History of Texas" (which occurred at a certain pharmacy school applied to by a friend from Texas, who attended college in another state). No one was denied medical school, because he or she studied world economics instead of U.S. economics or studied Christian literature instead of atheist literature, or vice versa.

Everyone had to take the Medical College Admission Test (MCAT), essentially the great equalizer.

All things being equal, they are not equal: I realize that sounds like something Yogi Berra would say. Fact is, wealth has its privileges, like a premier education since pre-school, the opportunity to choose an academic major on your interests rather than worrying about future employability, and having the financial means to afford specialized preparation courses for exams like the MCAT. All of those factors inherently give advantage toward admission to a professional school. It must be inherently less stressful to study for a final exam without having to simultaneously dart over to the Financial Aid Office to file forms and face the possible threat that your finances could fall short and all your effort only obtain half the step toward a degree and leave you smothered in debt.

The aforementioned debt is why a number of U.S. citizens forgo college. Susan M. Dynarski has wrote extensively regarding the availability of financial aid impacting enrollment and completion of higher education. Dynarski's 1999 "Does Aid Matter? Measuring the Effect of Student Aid on College Attendance and Completion" cites work by Larry Leslie and Paul Brinkman in 1988 indicating at that time a $1,000 decrease in tuition cost would increase college attendance between 3-5%. A more recent New York Times article by Susan Dynarski on September 20, 2014, indicated the apparent rise in tuition costs were due to shifting more of the education costs to the students with less portion from state (taxpayer) funds over time, but the actual revenue per student when adjusted for inflation is relatively flat over approximately the past 25 years. All I know is that when my uncles went to college in the late 1960s to early 1970s, they could work a summer job and save money for college, whereas in the early 1980s I was working most the year to afford one quarter of junior college.

Still, you must go on and even without wealth and preparatory courses. Ironically, although the MCAT weighs heavily on medical school admission criteria, it is not a predictor of success as a physician.

Chapter 4
Where Will You Go?

Most of those desiring to be a physician, a healer, are willing to study anywhere in the country, perhaps even anywhere in the world. In the United States, advanced education is usually managed via the individual states, which essentially means the only places you stand a chance of an interview is your home state. If one grows up in one state and attends college in another state, then the student has potentially two home states in reference to professional school applications. Some states have more medical schools than others. States without medical schools need arrangements with states that do have such programs, which creates its own logistic demographic distribution difficulties, like how many class slots are saved for people from certain states not having a medical program?

Then interview season arrives, and you have few interviews but no offers. A thought belatedly occurred to me – although quite proud that in the late 1990s I could still fit in the blue pinstripe suit from my 1982 Graduation from HVAC school, and proud of being frugal, the interviewers in the 1998-99 interview season only see an anachronism in his outdated suit. I had no cash to buy a new suit, but must have a new suit; prudence be damned, charge a new suit on credit – it's only more debt and miniscule to the amount of total student loan debt.

The answer to the ultimate question for a medical student applicant is not 42, but "Yes, I want to go into primary care." The question goes something along the lines of "Where do you see yourself in 5 or 10 years?" or "What field of medicine are you interested in?" Transplant surgery was a motivation for my interest in medical school during undergrad studies and making my interest in surgery known to medical school interviewers certainly weighed against me, because exactly as I was told by one undergraduate professor, "Medical school admissions personnel want to hear you are interested in primary care." Well, I could not lie, so I stated my interest in surgery and possibly transplant surgery and did not get accepted into some of those schools because of my honesty. My compromise was just to say, "I don't know," since I could not overtly lie and claim I had a motivation for a medical specialty I knew nothing about. I was not averse to family medicine; I just knew nothing about it. There were no doctors in my family to encourage me or discourage me in any particular medical specialty direction.

Finally, someone became interested, but their medical school class was already full and I was "Wait Listed," meaning placed on a list of potential candidates if others drop their candidacy from the program, typically by moving to their more preferred option. More Wait List letters arrive and one's heart sinks, but you keep faith. Place your faith in God, not man. Most people applying to medical school, or probably any form of higher education and graduate level programs, are not good at waiting; we are used to making things happen. One day, typically as you have already began making alternative plans, you get a call: "Would you like to enter our medical school?"

Dream fulfilled.

Part 2:

Medical School

Chapter 5
Medical School and Choosing
a Potential Residency

Typically, the first two years of medical training are spent in the classroom and another two years in clinic rotations. Getting used to a big transition – the workload in medical training – is incredible. When given a stack of notes the size of a large phone book, you are impressed with the amount of information there is to learn. When you suddenly realize that material was only for the first couple weeks and not the entire semester, you are petrified. In comparison, in undergraduate school one could review material the night before an exam, but in medical school a review must be started on a Friday evening and continue all weekend for a Monday morning exam.

Clinic experiences are sometimes like being in a clique, except you cannot leave if you do not fit in. Often your clinical experiences will guide you in choosing a medical specialty. The clinic years can make a lasting wonderful – or a horrible – impression. My choice of potential residency training changed several times and was based on personal interests and on observation for specialties in which I saw smiling residents or satisfied attending physicians, which were very few. Specialties like pathology, radiology, radiation oncology, dermatology, orthopedic surgery, occasionally family medicine and psychiatry, were of the few medical specialties where physicians smiled. When I saw a lot of miserable residents and mean bitter attending physicians, like in General Surgery and OB/GYN, I avoided those career selections.

Ironically, like the term "underrepresented minority," the term "primary care" is also politically malleable in that

OB/GYN is considered primary care regarding student loan interest, and debt reduction schemes, yet not really primary care as in the definition of general practice and probably not considered primary care to many medical school admissions personnel. Since I had prior experience troubleshooting and working with my hands in HVAC work, a specialty like OB/GYN, which required the intellectual application of medical knowledge combined with manual dexterity seemed like it would be a good fit for me. Unfortunately, although I would likely have found surgery and OB/GYN interesting, the abject misery of those specialties steered me away.

The typical surgery conversation was based upon malpractice issues and divorces. As if police officers and doctors in general did not have high enough suicide and divorce rates, I did not want a medical specialty that would make it inherently even more likely I would kill myself or get divorced.

There is so much litigation in obstetrics that many medical students avoid it like a plague. The sad reality is that any time something happens to a baby, someone gets punished and someone is compensated. A situation that used to be called "crib death" got re-named to sudden infant death syndrome (SIDS) and has landed some people in trouble with the legal system. SIDS will too often have some cloud of suspicion over the parents and imply failure of the medical personnel; such a situation attracts prosecutors trying to build a political career, malpractice lawyers looking for a potential big payoff, politicians posturing for votes and media circus most doctors want no part of. Even if the mother is an alcoholic crackhead who chain-smokes during the entire pregnancy and her abusive boyfriend regularly kicks her in the belly, if there is anything wrong with the kid, someone, like the driver of another vehicle in a tiny fender-bender accident in a parking lot, or the OB physician, will ultimately be sued. The abortion quagmire does not help attract people to the OB/GYN specialty either, as ending up libeled, slandered, under legal scrutiny, or feeling morally conflicted on a regular basis is not a life most honest law-abiding people with some sense of integrity and respect for life want to live. Not having the ideal doctors for a given specialty will only propagate the likelihood of medical errors, tragic outcomes and increase malpractice litigation, which is a vicious cycle.

I am reminded of a young woman presenting to the emergency department during my internship year for "vaginal bleeding." That was the complaint, not "I'm pregnant and have vaginal bleeding" or "I am so many month's pregnant, my OB doc is [place name here] and I have vaginal bleeding...nope, just vaginal bleeding." The Emergency attending physician and I walk into the room, and the young woman's belly is very large, like late-term pregnancy large. The attending physician states, "You're pregnant," and the young woman says, "No shit." The attending physician asks, "How far along are you?" The woman shrugs and says, with a combination of more than a little bit of bad attitude, apathy and irritation in her voice, "I don't know." So here is a young single pregnant woman with no idea of how far along in pregnancy she is, no history of any prenatal care, and has the serious pregnancy complication of late-term vaginal bleeding, which could represent something potentially catastrophic, and she does not seem to even care. If something goes wrong with the pregnancy and something bad happens to her or the baby, then she and her lawyer-to-be will suddenly care. As usual, the father-to-be is nowhere to be found for the young woman in the aforementioned condition, but I have no doubt if anything bad happened, he would materialize from out of nowhere to attempt to collect something in a lawsuit. Quick calls to OB doctors were made, and the patient rapidly transferred out of the general emergency room to an OB service. Of course, despite the lack of prenatal care and confrontational attitude of the patient against the very people trying to help her, possibly saving her life and the baby's life, if anything goes wrong the doctors will be sued, and the hospital and anyone else will be sued, too, just to cover all bases. There is no such thing as bad luck or personal accountability; the philosophy is to blame someone else, as it evidently pays well.

The honest fact is that pregnancy is not a totally benign condition. Historically, some small percent of women die in childbirth. Babies have died throughout mankind's existence and pregnancy complications happen; it's a sad fact of life. Efforts to decrease maternal and infant mortality in childbirth are to be lauded and have made improvements in many societies, but the risk is not zero. Such sad situations provide heart-wrenching drama that the media loves to exploit, there is substantial financial compensation available for such tragedies. This large financial compensation package is available even when there is no actual malpractice. Dr. De-Luca et al. in Lancet Neurology 2012; 11:283-92 have scientifically well-documented that other factors, much more than any medical negligence, cause cerebral palsy (CP). Their research cites many articles dating back to Dr. Little's statements in 1861, but most of the articles cited were from the past 25 years. De-Luca et al. indicate that around 30 years after Dr. William John Little wrote his impression relating CP to perinatal asphyxia, Sigmund Freud questioned Dr. Little's conclusions regarding the origin of CP. Yet even still, OB physicians are sued for Cerebral Palsy, especially if the malpractice insurance company choses to settle without ever going to court. I assure you that in court enough jurors are going to want to give something of someone else's money to compensate a young mother grieving on the witness stand. Even though science has proven most instances of CP are not the doctor's fault, no one is giving the money back or restoring doctors' reputations from all prior CP judgments.

Chapter 6
Honesty is Not Always the Best Policy

When going through mandatory medical school rotations, the correct answer to the question "What medical specialty are you interested in?" is whatever medical specialty you are on at the time. An OB/GYN resident took an immediate dislike to me simply because I answered that my favorite rotation to that point in time was orthopedic surgery. She immediately assimilated an agitated posture and quickly changed demeanor, like a cat being held too close to water. She went from apparently nice to instantly hostile over one moment. I sensed the attitude was, "Oh, orthopedics, you must think you are important and too good for us." She became quietly malignant towards me by not even telling me where or what time I should meet up with the team – then chastise me for being late; she subsequently also wrote terrible libel in my evaluation regarding my work ethic. I later learned many medical students' evaluations by the OB/GYN residents were essentially libelous as well. Evidently the medical student evaluation was the place for frustrated residents to vent, instead of confronting the supervisors who created and allowed such a malignant experience to exist.

During that rotation a woman with gestational diabetes felt dizzy on her way out of the bathroom, as I was passing by her room. Forgetting I was a lowly medical student and acting as a human being, I helped her back to a seat in her room and called the nurse. One of the OB/GYN residents saw me leaving the room and scolded me by stating, "What were you doing there? Those are private patients, you don't see them." Later, that same OB/GYN resident spent almost 15 minutes berating me for my diagnosis regarding a patient's postpartum situation, I did feel vindicated when the Maternal Fetal Medicine attending physician specialist agreed with my assessment. A few years after I had graduated medical school I heard that OB/GYN program had some of the few good attending physicians leave and the program was facing potential academic probation.

Surgical hierarchy is much like the military, and breaking the chain of command will get you in trouble and offending a superior has severe consequences. Offending a superior could be as simple as a medical student asking the senior resident if any particular salve, ointment or antibacterial is placed on a wound during your first day of surgery rotation. Seriously, one medical student asked such a question and was harassed the entire month on that service, including working until late in the evening before the shelf exam the next morning, then libeled in the evaluation by the statement, "Student cannot even change a Band-Aid." The student had to remediate a month of surgery rotation. Personally, I think the individual who was harassing the student and the administrator covering for such actions belonged in prison, not practicing medicine. As an aside: Many years prior to this episode, when I had surgery to remove a ganglion cyst on my finger, the plastic surgeon did recommend bacitracin daily on the wound. Not only would the bacitracin help fight infection, it apparently would prevent the sutures from sticking to the healing skin tissue and make a nicer healed wound appearance. Point is, the medical student's question was not out of line. I did write a letter of complaint regarding the abuse of my classmate, and my documentation was later raised as an indictment against me being a "troublemaker" during a meeting with a dean regarding a different breach by the medical school. So yes, in my experience everything you say and do in medical school, especially lodging a complaint, is saved by the deans/administrators to potentially be leveraged against you in the future, if needed.

Another medical student on surgery rotation got stuck with a needle by the attending surgeon during an operation. Following school policy and law in many states, the medical student reported the needle stick to student health as instructed. That student failed surgery and had to remediate a month. So, yes, there are those who use your honesty as a weapon against you. Obviously, neither of those medical students I mentioned went into surgery. Hence, those cases are examples of good, intelligent honest people being driven away from a certain medical specialty and also impacted those who knew them.

During one surgery, I saw a more senior medical student suddenly pull a finger back, and the attending asked "Did I get you?" meaning, "Did I stick you with the needle?" That medical student was interested in a surgery residency, so the student answered, "No." After all, a medical student who reports a needle stick is not likely to get a good recommendation for going into surgery residency.

The fact that the school administrators allowed such persecution to happen is appalling, but even more unfortunate is that such situations have become expected and accepted as part of the dehumanizing process of medicine training.

Chapter 7
Tainting the Evidence in
Evidence Based Medicine

Of note, the content in this chapter is from the first edition of this book self-published under the label Collimator Press in 2015 and is before open allegations about 'fake news' or the debate over scientific literature during the Covid-19 pandemic.

I learned how politically and financially motivated the concept of evidence-based medicine and medical research in America had become. Like most political propaganda, there was a nice name, but no real substance, so the opposite of the actual name was often true. The problem is that the concept of "evidence-based medicine" seems innately good and is now such Gospel that it has become public policy mantra and nests itself into the compliance and medico-legal/malpractice realm. This situation is a problem because much of the "evidence" in evidence-based medicine is based upon special interests, and some of the so called "evidence" had been outright fraud, like the rigged data provided to the FDA for a certain lipid lowering agent.

For example, over time a lot of propaganda and marketing was used to convince women in America that only barbarian and heathen native women breastfed their children. So at least an entire generation or more has been raised on bottle-feeding, instead of breastfeeding, which later in time is implicated to may have caused untold psychological stress upon said generation. It took a lot of fighting during several decades to even get the medical community to publicly acknowledge that breastfeeding was OK. Eventually, the medical community even became convinced breastfeeding was actually good – it worked for many thousands of generations of human existence 'til bottle-feeding came about, after all. Hence, breastfeeding became acceptable again, even recommended, for women in developed nations.

The pharmaceutical and baby food industries needed to do something to remain relevant in the baby nutrition supplement market. What better way to stay relevant than to create some "evidence"? During pediatrics rotation, we were given an article to read and discuss. The article was regarding iron supplementation in the setting of Physiologic Anemia of Infancy. The propaganda of the article was "ah-ha," breastfeeding is now OK, but not good enough. The idea was that for some reason it was necessary to have a pharmacologic battle against a normal physiologic process. Normal physiology of a developing child has a phase of growth imbalance whereby relative to body size and fluid volume the developing child is relatively anemic. Apparently, humanity throughout history has passed through this normal physiologic phase unscathed. No, this was not giving mom an iron supplement or a multivitamin to ensure she had adequate nutrients for herself and child, it was giving a supplement directly to the baby: essentially the situation was to market a solution to a nonexistent problem. Evidently, now modern pharmacy must fight normal physiology. Our professor seemed brainwashed by the mantra that this article was "evidence-based medicine," and thus as holy as the Word of God. Even when several astute students pointed out the fact that disclosures indicated the entire study was sponsored by a pharmaceutical company that provided iron nutrition supplement formula for babies and had a significant financial interest in the outcome, the professor was unwavering in his belief that this was legitimate evidence: Gospel. The article even overtly denied a well-known, well-documented fact that high medicinal doses of iron in the human gastrointestinal (GI) tract causes constipation in many, if not most people. The fact that almost everyone ever taking an iron supplement has often complained of associated constipation was completely ignored. The professor even acknowledged many of the parents of the infants given the iron supplementation complained the child developed constipation, but he believed that those parents must have been lying or imagining there was a problem, because this article said it was not a problem. So, if an article says something directly contrary to your own life experience, then you evidently did not experience it? Believe the article and deny reality. The issue of constipation was a statistically significant finding in the data "Results" of the article but was dismissed as insignificant in the "Discussion" component of the study and ignored in the "Conclusion" of the article. Sounds like the Amerasia scandal coverage described in "Blacklisted by History" – consider any objectionable findings as incidental, dismiss the objections as insignificant, and ignore everything not related to what you want known – also sounds like the more recent politics of Covid "science".

What to do when the "evidence" in evidence-based medicine is biased? What is worse is that an actual thinking physician practicing according to real world biology and physiology, instead of embracing propaganda presented as "evidence," is ridiculed by colleagues and open to persecution and malpractice litigation for not following the manipulated, financially-motivated propaganda as if it is Gospel. Seriously, long after medical school, a friend recently showed me an article forwarded from an MD Ph.D. friend of his regarding the fact that one of the cholesterol lowering drugs used fake data sent to the FDA for approval. A decade later, that data was proven as fraud.

Under President George W. Bush, Congress passed a law forbidding Americans from purchasing medications for a lower price in Canada, under the now proven false premise "those drugs are not FDA regulated, thus may not be safe." Yet we now see a regulated, very popular cholesterol-lowering medication given FDA approval based on fraud. Also, that inquisitive friend of mine showed me the countries of origin where his FDA-approved blood thinner medication came from, and it was not the United States. So, you cannot go buy a medication yourself from outside the United States, but the U.S. pharmacies can have your medication made overseas, shipped in, and given a hefty price mark-up and that is legal. My inquisitive friend's blood thinner medication was mostly made by compounding pharmacies in China and India. There were a couple places outside China and India making his medication, but none were in the United States. Ask yourself and ask your so-called 'representatives' in Congress and the Senate and White House, how can U.S. politicians forbid Americans from purchasing the same medication in Canada at a much lower price than the same medication in the United States, when none, or few, of the medications are even made in the Western hemisphere, let alone not made in the United States?

So, in this background of real science and medicine and trying to do the right thing, there are a lot of lies and deception. How do you know what is true or not? Fact is, in school you are tested on memorizing so-called knowledge, regardless if most of the "knowledge" you memorize is a lie. It sounds like the Weird Al Yankovic song "Everything You Know is Wrong."

Chapter 8
Shelf and STEP Examinations

One stressful part of clinical rotations was the national shelf examination at the end of each rotation. The national shelf exam is mostly designed to give an indication how students individually and how students of an academic institution in general compare against the national average. Such information can be used to show strengths and weaknesses in training by institutions and of individuals, which can lead to educational improvement. Although the exam agency specifically states, "it is not recommended to use these test scores for the final class evaluation," my school utilized the shelf exam scores for the final class evaluation. In talking to students from other schools, I learned many schools used the shelf exams for grading analysis, despite a stated contraindication by the examining agency. The more troubling part is we never saw our actual exam score result directly from the testing agency. Thus, it is conceivable a professor could contrive any score results for the shelf exam and you had no way to confirm or refute the results.

All medical students who want to practice medicine in the United State eventually will take the United States Medical Licensing Exam (USMLE) sequence in three steps. USMLE Step 1 is typically taken after second year of medical school, prior to your clinical rotation years. For most medical students the entire future medical career opportunities depended on your USMLE Step 1 score. Of course, no one from school administration tells you that your future medical career solely based upon the USMLE Step 1 score, because people who do exceptionally well on Step 1 tend to go into medical specialties, whereas those doing more average or on the lower side of average are steered into primary care. Since there is a big push to get more medical students to enter a primary care career, it behooves the school to have people pass Step 1, but not have too many students do so extraordinarily well on Step 1 that they all go into specialty fields. Also, if you are an MD/Ph.D. student, youy really good or even great Step 1 score at the time you took the exam could end up being an average score when compared to future exam results when you are completing your Ph.D. work, clinical years, and applying to residency programs.

The aforementioned situation where your great exam score value today is an average score result compared to exams taken in the future is called Grade Creep. Since the average board exam score tends to increase over time, comparing a score result of an exam taken several years ago to those taken presently are inherently skewed against the person taking the exam several years earlier, which helps limit people from leaving primary care and reapplying to a different specialty at a later time. You would like to think your other skills, interests, research accomplishments and grades make a difference, too, but many residency programs make their first cut based solely in the Step 1 score.

Part 3:

Transition from Medical School to Residency and Becoming a Physician

Chapter 9
More Examinations

Before you graduate medical school, you usually take USMLE Step 2 (Step 2). Generally, you squeeze your Step 2 exam during your lighter clinical rotations, during elective rotations or during any breaks you may have. In medicine, studying for and taking a national exam is considered a "break." Go figure.

Eventually, after you graduate medical school, during internship year or the following year, you take the USMLE Step 3 exam and are then eligible to apply to be a licensed physician. Later in training or after completing residency training, you take your specialty board exams.

Unfortunately, every 10 years you have to keep taking your specialty boards or participate in a board longitudinal assessment program for life; I suspect it is purely a money-making scheme for the specialty boards, because if you practice your medical specialty every day over many years and take 50 to 100 continuing medical education (CME) credits every year or two, there is no logical reason for ever taking a recertification exam or additional assessments. I understand recertifying if you have been away from the field for some time, but otherwise there is no legitimate reason for having to recertify. Also, when setting up these specialty board recertification exams, those developing the scheme managed to exempt themselves from the recertification process via "grandfather clauses." If the people creating the recertification schemes really believed recertification was necessary and vitally important for optimal patient care, they would have practiced what they preached and not exempted themselves from the system they created.

Like most of politics, when rules have significant exemptions, maybe it is not a good rule to begin with?

Chapter 10
Residency MATCH

When applying for a medical residency, there is a "Match" system. In theory, the process begins when you send your information to programs for the medical specialty or specialties in which you are interested, then you get some interviews and match into the best fit for you. In reality, there are a limited number of government determined residency openings/slots/positions in any given year for each medical specialty at each institution. The limited number of residency position openings is often arbitrary and more often politically motivated and determined by the Center for Medicare and Medicaid Services (CMS): Don't ask me why it is not CMMS, because it appears apparently many government and medical acronyms do not follow the rules for their abbreviation formation. CMS uses taxpayer money to fund residency positions. Since most hospitals want money they take on residents to get in on the financial action. No one actually gives financial information to medical students and residents, it is more of a "sign here policy." Obtaining a straight answer to a simple question such as, how much does an institution receive in funding per resident is impossible? The government calculations are convoluted and involve direct and indirect sources of funding, which are adjusted by political debate, special interest lobbying and toying with definition of underserved populations and underserved regions. So much for government transparency to the taxpayer. In her 2012 health policy fellowship presentation "The Future of Graduate Medical Education Funding," Kimberly A. Hopely stated there are about 111,000 students in residency for a given year and about $9.5 billion in CMS funding, which translates to approximately $86,000 per resident in 2009 dollars. Given that a 2014 residency salary range varies from approximately $45,000 to $55,000 that situation at first glance leaves around $30,000 per resident going into the coffers of training institutions, which can add up to a lot of money. Small wonder many medical school administrators and college administrators make a lot more money than actual practicing physicians. But, that additional money comes with a myriad of conditions, documentation and compliance requirements. Also, government funding for a given resident is based on the specialty matched in, not the specialty desired. For example, if you applied for Radiology and had five years of funding potentially allotted, but matched into Family Medicine, then you are funded for only three years. Any further residency training on your part is financially on you, the institution hiring you, or a sponsor. For some places, that difference between a resident's salary and the funding amount is a financial windfall, while some break even, and some even determine the economics of supporting residency programs in the age of hyper-regulation are not worth the effort.

When you consider that medical residents needed legislation to reduce work hours to only 80 hours per week, not counting exceptions to the rule, you notice the income of $50,000 at an 80- hour work week, minus vacation time equals about $13/hr. for someone with four years or more of education plus on-the-job training after college. When you find the average construction laborer salary in the United States on Payscale.com during that same time period is approximately $13.72, you realize medical residents are a bargain at that price. Do not forget that medical residents will pay federal, state and in many cases local income taxes. Thus, a significant amount of the money paid out in medical resident training expenses comes back to the government in the form of tax revenue, so the cost of medical resident training is less than it initially appears. Some people like myself who have changed residencies after not matching into the desired field were no longer funded positions, which means the costs of training are not directly supported by the government: hence, an even better deal for the government and taxpayers. Ms. Hopely's numbers indicate an incidence of about 22,000 residency positions annually and a prevalence of around 111,000 medical residents in any given year, which indicates a five-year average funding for residency training across the board. Thus, if someone wanted to decrease the residency training budget, lowering the residency terms would help. How much training is necessary, versus how much is relatively cheap labor? Seriously, if nurse practitioners and physician assistants who have less training than a medical student are allowed to take over many duties once performed by physicians, how many years of residency on-the-job training are really required past medical school in most instances? With the appropriate budgetary flexibility residents could get their experience numbers while shaving a year or more off training. For example, surgery residents on some of the medical missions I have attended performed more thyroid surgeries in one week on the mission than in their five years of residency in a United States program. We can get those residents such experience not only on overseas missions work, but right here in America, but it requires a training budget system designed to allow such flexibility. Since the whole residency system is all about money and power brokering, limiting the number of residency positions funded at any given institution and limiting the number of funded positions for any given medical specialty residencies leads to strong government influence in the number of people allowed to train and practice in any given region and any given specialty, totally independent of actual population needs. If, from my explanation, the medical residency system appears a lot like a Stalin Command Society model, it is. If the medical residency system sounds like a bad way to allocate highly educated and highly skilled personnel resources to fill the needs of society, it is.

There was a lawsuit against the monopoly Match system, but then I heard nothing more about it. Years later, perusing a radiology journal, I stumbled across an article addressing why a legal battle against perceived unfair government reimbursement schemes was not likely to succeed due to legal precedents regarding the unquestionability of CMS payment decisions. The author of this radiology article also mentioned the lost lawsuit against the U.S. residency Match program as an example. During an active lawsuit, Congress intervened to change the rule of law by adding an unrelated rider onto an overwhelmingly approved pension law. The lawsuit against the Match system began in 2002 and The Pension Funding Equity Act, PUBLIC LAW 108–218—APR. 10, 2004 SEC. 207. CONFIRMATION OF ANTITRUST STATUS OF GRADUATE MEDICAL RESIDENT MATCHING PROGRAMS added to the end of the pension act assured monopoly status and antitrust immunity for the MATCH system: "(c) EFFECTIVE DATE.—This section shall take effect on the date of enactment of this Act, shall apply to conduct whether it occurs ***prior to*** [emphasis added], on, or after such date of enactment, and shall apply to all judicial and administrative actions or other proceedings pending on such date of enactment." Case dismissed.

Hopefully you can see the serious problem of laws with retroactive scope, and am terrified that such a concept can even exist in a so-called free society or any society of laws. For those who don't understand the significance of retroactive scope laws, it means the rules of law you follow today, can be completely disregarded or overturned at a later date and that future law can be used to prosecute you for past actions that were once perfectly legal. Essentially, such manipulation of the law means the rule of law has no sustainable foundation. Also, the fact that 'riders' are allowed means many laws are not passed on their true merit, but on political manipulation, which further erodes any foundation for the formation of laws of a society. A situation where a law is not evaluated on its individual merit undermines the concept of Democracy or Representative Republic, because riders take the individual review process away from the legislators by bundling laws in a batch, and take away the ability of the voters to hold a given representative accountable for any specific law by blending popular and objectionable legislation together. More examples of damage caused by Riders will be seen later.

When you realize people went to jail (i.e. "Club Fed") for violating insider trading laws that Congress had exempted itself from, you will not be so surprised at all regarding Congress' involvement in the lawsuit against the Match and realize we essentially have two classes in America – a political class and the rest of the country that funds the political class.

Here is the situation regarding the Match process. Choosing a medical field of focus takes a lot of introspective soul searching. You are choosing a field of medical practice you expect to be in the rest of your life and the training for that medical focus will take anywhere from about three to ten years or more, it is no small commitment. Yes, actually even the "general practice"/ "primary care" fields like general internal medicine, family medicine, pediatrics and obstetrics/gynecology are examples of still somewhat of a specialty focus.

Suppose you really like a competitive medical specialty. Competitive specialty means you need someone lobbying for your admission. For example, there are many potential great dermatologists out there in medical school, but dermatology is a competitive residency with relatively very few slots compared to other residencies. The outcome has been that in many parts of the nation there is over a six-month wait to see a dermatologist, which may be inconvenient for some skin conditions, but can be deadly in the case of melanoma. I actually read a clinic note documenting a situation where the patient's yet-to-be diagnosed melanoma grew significantly during the wait to see a dermatologist. Since that patient had metastatic disease at initial diagnostic work-up at a cancer facility it is very plausible it metastasized during the treatment delay. That case is at least one example witnessed by this one doctor, where the U.S. government communist command society model restricting the number of dermatologists has caused a death, as survival rates for metastatic malignant melanoma are low.

Chapter 11
Wage Economics, a Sad Story
for Many Americans

On the other end of the residency spectrum, away from the highly specialized medical tracks are medical fields like general internal medicine, family medicine, pediatric and medicine/pediatrics combined programs. In theory at least, specialists can practice in general medicine fields they trained in prior to specializing, but general practitioners are not typically able to practice in a specialty field. The point is, that although government funding is manipulated to favor more general practice sorts of positions and to discourage a large number of specialty positions, the economic factors, malpractice environment, and lifestyle leads people into more specialized medical fields or carving out some sort of specialty niche, versus leaving medicine altogether. For example, my recollection of a Money Magazine article in the 1980s stated that the average income for a Family Medicine physician was about $105,000 to $115,000 annual salary, whereas by 2010 the average Family Medicine physician salary was in the $125,000 to $135,000 annual salary range. According to the Government Accounting Office July 1986 report, table 3, the net pre-tax income of Internal Medicine physicians in 1984 was a mean of approximately $103,000 in an AMA survey and approximately $90,000 in the Medical Economics survey. Deriving the rate from the simple interest formula I=P*r*t yields a rate = I/(P*t). Comparing the change in income between $90,000 in 1984 and $135,000 in 2010 gives an approximate 1.9% annual raise on the high end, whereas the change between $103,000 in 1984 and $125,000 in 2010 yields 0.82% annual raise in salary. Average annual inflation calculated over that same

26-year period was about 2.9% and the cost of living was lower and portion of income gone to taxes was lower in the 1980s than 2010. Such a situation means that physicians' salaries have relatively fallen approximately 1-2% per year compared to inflation, much like the relative income for jobs in many industries had fallen compared to about 1979 levels. As an example of the general dire employment salary situation in the United States, I remember some of the guys in high school earning about $10/hr. doing landscaping in the late 1970s and early 1980s; that same job in 2012 paid about $8/hr. and had no benefits. Grocery clerk and cashier jobs used to be a career, but since about 1983, the top rate for new hires at a grocery store where I used to work dropped significantly under a split-tier system, and those jobs now may not have benefits. I heard of a general surgeon in the 1970s who worked very hard and made around a million dollars in a certain year; by comparison, in a few decades later a general surgeon's salary is about a third of that value. Not only has the training cost gone up while salaries have dropped, the cost of malpractice has soared and all other costs of doing business have increased. Hence, essentially until the Trump presidency, in several industries, including medicine, wages have fallen absolutely, relatively, or both compared to inflation.

Couple the absolute and relative decrease in physician salaries with the enormous bone crushing student loan debt burden, and you can see problems on the horizon. For example, I have had physicians tell me of their student loan debt in the 1980s being around $20,000, which was near or even well below the median income for a family of four in the United States at that time. Now, almost $300,000 in student loan debt is not all that unusual, and $150,000 student loan debt for the average physician is quite typical; mine was about $250,000 with a good chunk of the money being interest accumulated during training and recapitulation of that interest into principal at time of repayment. Unlike a certain recent Secretary of State who managed to pay off about $24 million of campaign debt with a $361,000 annual gross income job, most of us doctors do not have such magic political accounting to alleviate our debt. Not being politicians, our numbers have to actually add up. The Tax Committee had not helped working Americans either. The tax deduction for student loan interest is phased out based on income level, which means most physicians do not get to deduct their student loan interest from their income taxes. Income averaging is also long gone, so there's no way to average those years of no income and low income against a sudden increase in salary after training. Many of us also do not get to deduct anything from income taxes, except charitable contributions, because Alternative Minimum Tax (AMT, the "millionaire tax" of the late 1960s never indexed to inflation) kicks in to essentially negate all your tax deductions and raise your federal tax rate: The 2017 tax bill amended the AMT threshold.

To further put physician income in perspective, in 2003 the average pediatrician salary was around $90,000 and at that time the Longshoremen union workers were making more than $100,000 annual income and went on strike for higher wages and better benefits. Thus, when you compare time spent, efforts exhausted, student loan debt, academic accomplishment, lifestyle sacrifices etc., many physicians are worse off to financially on par with well-paid unskilled union labor. The whole situation gives a sad idea of how little American society values education in general and its physicians in particular. Of course, in the current social climate people find it popular to demonize the salary of hard-working business leaders and doctors, while no complaints are levied regarding the exorbitant salaries of celebrities and athletes, or the ability of politicians to live well beyond the means of their published salaries.

Chapter 12
Student Loans

My advice is to keep student loan payment records for life and have them buried with you in the casket – not exactly the Pharaoh's treasure, but if you are exhumed and your body interrogated for something of value to the government, you can show compliance and future grave robbers can see what current society values. Sarcasm aside, I found out the hard way about not having old student loan documents. I had attended trade school and was in HVAC a decade before going back to college full time and subsequent medical training. I had long paid my trade school student loan debts and the school and government always had my contact information.

Approaching my last year of medical school, I received a letter demanding about $500 for an unpaid portion of my trade school student loan. I did remember a grant for about $530, and my understanding was grants did not need to be paid back and so had no idea where this $500 demand suddenly came from. I was certain there must have been some mistake and was sure I paid everything off about 15 years prior to the letter arriving. When the trade school I long ago attended closed down, auditors went into the school computers and claimed to have found unpaid loans or portions of unpaid loans. When threatened by the student loan debt situation in question, I immediately went to my bank and credit union of the time looking for my account transaction data. There was no record of those payments. A representative explained to me that banks and credit unions kept records in compliance with tax regulations, for seven years. Hence, they had no way to give me detailed information from my former account activities 15 years ago and earlier. After selling my house, going to college full time, moving to a different city for medical school etc., I culled a lot of documents I thought no longer mattered. I know I paid my trade school loans off completely, long before that letter arrived, but had no way to prove it. I had no means to double-check the auditors and was surviving off student loans. I was at a vulnerable time needing more student loans for the last year of medical school and living on Ramen noodles with a can of mixed vegetables added, which is not a position of strength to initiate a challenge against government auditors. I did formally complain to the ombudsman about the ancient debt, the likely error, and the impossibility of getting old bank statements to prove my case. Some downward adjustment to the bill was made, but I still paid most of the contested amount out of my medical school student loan allocation and cut back on meal budget for the semester (no vegetables for the Ramen noodles). Student loans are for life, but the banking documents showing your payments of student loans are only kept for a relatively few years. Sadly ironic is the fact the FBI and NSA can have records of every citizen of America and many leaders the world and probably have every transaction I ever made dating back to kindergarten, yet such resources are not accessible to benefit a citizen, only to prosecute or persecute someone. Therefore, my advice is keep many copies of any student loan repayment proof in many forms, because if there is ever any problem, it is your task to prove innocence. Congress could very simply enact a law that banks had to hold financial records, at least student loan payment records, for 30 years or 50 years or make some sort of statute of limitations on resurrecting old debt, but I will not hold my breath.

Part 4:

Internship and Residency

Chapter 13
Internship

Internship is hell, and there is no nicer way to describe it. Internship is like a bleak darkness you are trying to paint on a black canvass and you cannot paint it black enough. Unfortunately, that image is the good side of internship. I did not work the consistent more than 100-hours work week as the system was in the days "House of God" was written but endured Internship during the changeover to making an 80-hour work week, with several exceptions and exemptions to allow longer work hours. The end result was a mad frenzy to perform the well over 100 hours of work within 80 hours. In the "old days," medical notes could be quite brief and much communication occurred verbally; now everything has to be documented, or it never happened. For example, a radiologist was successfully sued because even though he provided appropriate patient care and appropriate communication to the treating physician, he did not document the communication – therefore it never happened, even though the subsequent actions taken by the treating physician physically proved appropriate communication had occurred. The lack of documentation on the part of the radiologist was interpreted by the plaintiff lawyer as a breach of recommended guidelines, and hence a breach in patient care. In the old days a doctor could see a patient for half an hour or more and document a five-minute or shorter note. Now the situation is reversed and doctors see a patient for under five minutes and have to write a 30-minute note. Hence, the fallout of extensive malpractice litigation and government compliance is that physicians actually spend more time documenting a patient encounter than actually encountering a patient. This situation has turned the physician role into a harried secretarial role, which means intelligence and critical analysis are little valued in medicine, only your speed of documentation matters. Politicians do not seem to realize the impossibility of lowering healthcare costs by legislating more rigorous documentation standards and ignore or deny the fact that physician perseveration on documentation, malpractice and compliance inherently takes the focus away from the patient.

By the way, some surgical residents at many programs did, and likely still do, work more than 120 hours per week but just document 80 hours. As indicated earlier, honesty is not always the best policy, especially if you want to avoid harassment. No surgery resident wants to be considered "weak" and "lacking commitment." Having mentors see you as weak is not good for your future. Thus, the future need of strong recommendation letters trumps integrity, regulatory compliance and personal health. The situation of working well over the 80 hours guidelines can happen in medicine training as well. To obtain a desirable medical subspecialty fellowship, you must impress your superiors. How better to impress than to apparently get over 100 hours a work accomplished much quicker than other residents? So, having a medicine intern working more than100 hours a week and documenting 80 hours a week or less did happen on occasion. During the time "House of God" was written, one year of internship was all that was required for you to be a general medicine practitioner. Now primary care general medicine, family medicine and pediatrics are three-year residencies and many fellowships are several additional years, instead of one additional year. Thus, although the Internship itself now has shorter workweek hours (still twice the average workweek hours in society), additional years have been added onto residency and fellowship training for medical specialties.

During internship, you would work call shifts limited to 30 hours. Yes, you came into the hospital and did not leave for the next 30 hours. During that time, you will desire sleep but get no sleep. Once evening strikes, there are only a few medical interns and a couple senior residents to cover the entire hospital. If you do attempt to sleep, you will be awoken every few minutes, which is against the Geneva Convention to do to a prisoner of war.

When you take some of the most humanitarian-minded people who have dedicated their lives to caring for others and subject them to the tortures of medical training, which are too abusive to do to "enemy combatants" and those training in military special services, you can expect to lose some of those characteristics so cherished in good physicians. Literally, the appreciation of life and compassion for ourselves and others has been driven out of us. We become a shell of the person we once were and slip into survival mode.

In Internship, survival is half the battle, not just for the patients, but for the intern as well. From the start of my first 4 a.m. shift the first day of Internship, I wondered "What have you done? You should have been a banker, they are still asleep!" I can only describe the year as one of cyclothymic disorder, where one is chronically depressed but not to the degree to be diagnosed with full depression. I was miserable and thought it was just me, until one of my seemingly well-adjusted colleagues indicated post-call, he would "go home, have some Gatorade to wash down a Zoloft (an anti-depressant) and get some sleep." The book "House of God" indicated that the most seemingly well-adjusted among the resident characters were either pretending to be happier than they were or being self-medicated for depression and anxiety. I used to cross a railroad track every day on my drive into work, and I frequently wished a train would take me away, but alas, the tracks were of a seasonal railway, mostly of historic significance to a bygone era and ran on daytime hours and summer weekends. I also wondered if I would fight or thank someone if they tried to kill me in the parking lot of our urban located hospital. Certainly, violence against me was possible in an outdoor, unguarded inner-city parking lot. Turns out, I was not alone in such sad thoughts.

Chapter 14
Historical Perspective on Residency

The idea of "residents" constantly in the hospital is based on an antiquated model of healthcare, which is around 100 years old. The residency concept was based upon seeing everything that came through the door of the hospital, as the residents and nurses did everything at that time. Patients were treated without three to five layers of bureaucracy trying to focus on ways to meet compliance and to get paid. The focus was on the patient and their disease; now the focus is on documentation and compliance. Since that older time, we have developed a healthcare system with transplant centers, cancer institutes, cardiac facilities, orthopedic surgical sites, etc. The point is that these days the medical system is more fragmented based upon patient medical diagnosis or organ system. Thus, you are never going to learn transplant surgery at a cancer hospital or a rural clinic. You will not develop trauma skills at a cancer institute, because you just will not see that patient population. Hence, that old residency model of physician training may have been appropriate in a different era, but is almost completely useless under the current medical practice paradigm. In fact, these days, a business background, legal acumen or chanting the appropriate political mantra is much more important than any scientific skills or medical knowledge, which should give you an idea how far medical care has gone in the wrong direction.

The other thing to remember about medical residency, especially Internship, is that entrenched attitude took till until about 1999 for the combination of all the medical resident suicides, post-call driving accident deaths, and medical errors to get some impetus for change and until about 2004 to finally get some refinements. In sad reality, mostly only the medical errors motivated change. There were a few lawsuits by family members that challenged the tradition of driving accidents and suicides being acceptable risk factors in residency, but for the most part medical errors were the causative agent for change. If the residents could have simply died without making medical mistakes affecting patients' lives, there would have been no change. Make no mistake, many attending physicians are bitter from their own experiences and wish the same abuse for current residents. We call such people "vindictive"; we also call them "the people in charge" of most of the medical education system. When I was in medical school, an Internal Medicine resident asked the then AMA president touring the various schools about residency hour restrictions, and he (a surgeon) made it quite clear he was opposed to any efforts at humane working conditions for residents. So yes, it took many deaths and lots of medical errors and much lobbying to get an 80-hour work week (no overtime pay), 30-hour call shifts and four days off per month (a day off being defined as any 24-hour time period). So yes, leaving work from an overnight call shift at 7 a.m. on a Friday and coming back to work at 7 a.m. Saturday morning was "a day off" – Ideally you got four of those a month.

There were also a myriad of exemptions to the rules, so residents could work about 100 hours and have 36-hour call shifts in the name of "continuity of patient care" if required. Since the time of the initial writing, a change has been made and the 80-hour limit rescinded for those classified as Interns and only counts for Residents. Those who challenged the system were blackballed as weak, troublemakers or idiots. So that idea of leaving work on a Friday afternoon and returning Monday morning that many people are so accustomed to was non-existent to quite rare in medicine and referred to as a "golden weekend," meaning the same thing most people referred to as a "weekend."

59

Chapter 15
The Question of No-Call

Some programs lured residents by offering protected time, like no-call months or research time, but later reneged on the "promise," using the term "promise" lightly, more in the "bait and switch" connotation of the word "promise." Below is an email regarding an issue apparently raised by some residents about an alleged promise of one month of no call:

Hello Everyone,

This topic has come up a few times for the interns so I'm just sending it out to you all.

I'm not sure where people got this idea but a few (and I do mean more than one) of you have suggested to me that it was in their contract (or at least somehow promised) to get at least one month of no call. There is nothing like that in your contract as far as I know nor are the directors aware of any such promise. Now, (---) and I do try and give interns on Core Electives No MORE than ONE call and NONE if POSSIBLE but you have to keep in mind that in doing that for you we SCREW someone else just so you can have no call instead of one which I really don't see as being that different. If you have any concerns or information of which I am not aware or feel that your call has been excessive feel free to meet with me. I can bring up exactly how many calls each of you have had over the year including how many weekends. The call scheduler can even calculate a score for each of you if you are really that concerned. However, let me just say that it's been pretty even

*between categoricals, prelims, and transitionals
(believe it or not). Please let me know of any
concerns and I'll do my best to resolve this issue
for you.*

*Thanks,
(---)*

I guess the program is implying that many residents evidently had "shared delusions" of a promise or implication that never happened.

Education programs inherently have a constant flux of new trainees, whereas administrators are fixed for a much longer time period. Little to no communication regarding prior promises or abuses is conveyed across the old and newer in-training population.

Hence, under the education umbrella, promises can easily be made and broken routinely, because new people do not know of former promises, broken promises or abuse, and those leaving are gone before the new ones arrive.

Chapter 16
One Bad Apple Can Spoil the Whole System: Forced to Tolerate the Intolerable

Fortunately, the person in the following example is not representative of most nurses, but unfortunately went into nursing for reasons other than patient care. When you have a nurse who does not follow orders all day then at the end of the shift suddenly decides to rush everyone through so she can leave on time or a little early it is a problem. One such nurse I had the displeasure of working with (if you can call her "working") was in the Emergency Department/ Emergency Room (ED aka ER). When I was there and she was supposed to be my nurse, I seldom saw her; my patients seldom saw her either. For example, all female pelvic exams performed by a male doctor required a female in the room, typically a female nurse. Many was the time a woman was waiting far too long for me to do a simple few minutes pelvic exam, because I had to wait for this poor excuse for a nurse to become available. I did not even need her to assist, just to show up. Simple orders, like administering a pill, never got done.

We had a patient with history of heart issues and wound complications from surgery leading to a part of the sternum (breast bone) being removed. When one breathes, the diaphragm muscles get innervated and are signaled to contract. The contracting of this convex parachute-like muscle causes it to flatten out. Simultaneously, the accessory muscles of respiration, like intercostal muscles (the muscles between the ribs) and the scalene muscles (muscles from the neck to the upper ribs) are activated. The muscles of respiration help enlarge the chest (aka thoracic cavity). The action of the breathing muscles (diaphragm and accessory muscles) makes a larger volume, thus decreases the intrathoracic pressure (decreases pressure within the chest). The decrease in intrathoracic pressure allows the lungs to expand and one can take a breath in. Relaxing of respiratory muscles and the spring-like resiliency inherent in normal, non-smoker, lungs, causes the lungs to passively contract and we exhale. Well, when someone is missing a structural bone element of the chest, like having ribs broken at two points or resection of a portion of the sternum, they get that unsupported area sucking in when inhaling and bulging out on exhalation, which is termed flail chest. Hence, when a constrictor snake crushes a victim's ribcage, there is no structural support to allow the lungs to expand, because instead the crushed ribs and unsupported skin of the thorax just sucks in. No lung expansion and contraction equals no breathing, which in short order yields death. So, when this patient was having unsettling symptoms it was worth investigating for recurrence of a heart situation or a result in a change of respiratory dynamics due to prior surgery. Also, besides already being anxious from breathing difficulty, the patient had a lot of bad things going on in life, so pressure and anxiety were also high in the differential. My attending physician leaned pretty heavily in the anxiety diagnosis and wanted me to prescribe an anxiolytic (typically a benzodiazepine [benzo in medical jargon and in street lingo], such as valium or Ativan).

Well, after many instances of talking with the aforementioned nurse and talking with pharmacy it became evident that after four hours, the medical order for a regularly-stocked medication like Ativan was never requested and processed by the nurse to be sent up from pharmacy. In other words, an imperative medical order for patient care, was willfully ignored for hours due to a negligent nurse and there was nothing I could do about it. Talk about a waste of patient's time – four hours to get a pill to swallow and go home. Meanwhile, other patients were waiting to be seen, while an ER bed is tied up several hours due to a bad nurse who belonged anywhere except in patient care (My tongue-in-cheek suggestions for prison or firing squad were, of course, ignored.). I was upset that my attempt to formally complain to the attending ED physicians was just ignored. Such a situation just lets you realize how powerless an intern is, even a doctorate level intern.

Later, when I was on a medicine team admitting patients through the ED, this same nurse wrenched a chart out of a doctor's hand to submit the admit orders. Finally, much later in the year, my last night of admitting call ever in medicine (thank God), that same nurse, evidently still with no reprimands, asked if we on the medical team planned to admit a certain patient or not; I stated "We needed to present the case to our attending physician." The nurse filled in the admission order, submitted it herself and the patient was sent out of the ED and to an inpatient room. That action was dangerous as the orders were not reviewed by the supervising physician, and an error or omission could have occurred placing the patient's life in jeopardy. I complained again to more senior residents, ED attending physicians and the medicine attending, but still to no avail – evidently, they too, felt powerless.

There are procedures built into the medical system to minimize errors and to save lives, but this nurse just bypassed those safeguards with impunity. To make matters legally worse, in certain states, like Ohio, you do not need a bad outcome for malpractice, just an "increased risk" of bad outcome is enough to sue and win. Obviously, a nurse bypassing safety steps to go home early after being lazy and belligerent all day is causing blatant increase in risk of patient harm every day. Essentially, by Ohio law, every patient ever seen anywhere when that nurse was working met the qualifications for a malpractice lawsuit victory based upon "increased risk of a bad outcome," I honestly do not know if that particular nurse was ever reprimanded or not and if her overt negligence ever cost the hospital a lawsuit or not, but the experience of having to protect patients from negligent staff and the feeling of being alone in that struggle leaves a lasting bitterness.

Chapter 17
New Nurses and Getting Orders Right

Most people may not know the significance of having unsigned orders in the chart. There are whole departments dedicated to nothing but making sure charts are signed. Of course, if doctors were not so pressed for time, such a department would be small and the need to catch minor oversights would be rare. One significance of an unsigned order is whether a doctor actually placed an order in the first place, especially if something ever went wrong and the merit of the order called into question. If orders are not signed, it can also be bad because the medical chart is legally discoverable evidence, and even the most mundane things can be contrived, by an attorney having the advantage of retrospective review, into a conspiracy or deemed to reflect negligence. Hence, many is the time doctors will be paged, emailed or called by phone to come to medical records and sign the unsigned orders. Being called to sign orders that are not yours is a nuisance, which is made more stressful because you are tracked and judged on how many and how long you have unsigned orders hanging out. It is understandably a stressful situation where you get demerits, threat of pay being withheld or administrative action against you for delay in signing an order that you did not even make. Also, unsigned orders can affect the ability for the hospital to get paid. There is an etiquette when various services are involved in patient care as to who actually writes the orders in the chart. For example, often a consulting service will make recommendations but rely on the primary service to execute the recommendations (Primary service writes the orders.). Having a lowly intern make an order that overrides a highly trained and seasoned specialist, or the primary service knowing the patient best, is not only absurd but appears quite rude as well.

Here is a sample of my email correspondence about nurses not documenting orders correctly and making a non-order into an apparent order. This event was shortly before end of internship year:

(---),

Tonight (earlier in the evening around 6pm) I received a call from a nurse regarding a patient in (---). She stated the cardiologist had called and said the echo was OK. I thought, so what? I told her no one signed out the patient to me, so I had no real reply to the information. She asked if the patient should stay on tele (telemetry unit).

Let me repeat that: the nurse, not the cardiologist, not the PCP, inferred the news from the cardiologist would exclude the patient from tele.

I stated that since I knew nothing of the significance of the results to the plan for this patient she should not change anything until the primary service views the results.

Later, on call (around 4:30 am) while seeing a different patient I went to see the chart on (---). Under the Orders Section I found the order "OK for Patient to continue telemetry, T.O. Dr Gannon."

I never gave that order. I don't think telling a nurse to stick with the current plan is a New Order. In effect a Secret Order, unknown by the physician he or she is giving an order. Such orders, can jeopardize a patient's health and create animosity among staff thinking residents are managing patients contradictory to the attending's plan.

It seems that this month there are a lot of new nurses and I get a lot of pages asking for interpretation of obvious orders or nurses questioning the plan of the primary service, such as deciding whether or not to discharge a patient (like today (---) after the PCP has already ordered the discharge. I have to check if that nurse wrote her decision as an order from me.

I will no longer have to deal with the issue here, but I still think the problem is serious and needs to be addressed.

Of course, in July, the seasoned nurses will have analogous issues when the new residents arrive.

Chapter 18
Getting Slammed on Call

Sometimes on call you get a lot of pages from one floor. The pagers stopped displaying more than 20 pages, but I know at least once I counted at least 28 calls. I think the display limit is to keep residents from getting any more depressed than they already are.

Typically, when on call, you are responsible for the lives of 120-150 people you never met, so it is really difficult to predict who will crash.

The biggest time-consuming issue when on call is a "family wants to talk to a doctor about plans for their (mother, sister, brother, etc.)." Patients or patients' families wanting to talk with doctors about patient care, is not inherently a nuisance, but made a nuisance by the fact that as the intern covering the entire hospital or a significantly large portion of the hospital patient population at any given time means you already are sleep deprived and have at least a few other urgent things you are supposed to be doing rather than talking to a family about a patient you know absolutely nothing about – talk about a "cram study session" under bad circumstances. The on-call doc seldom knows any of the patients as he or she may not even be working in the hospital that month, so having a doctor who does not know about a patient talk to family is often a waste of everyone's time. Apparently, nurses have been instructed to contact the on-call intern rather than bother the actual treating physician who knows the patient and plan of care. Occasionally you subsequently even find out the family members lied when they said the "regular physician was unavailable," because you talk with a physician who knows that patient and find out that three people tried several times to get in contact with family members over several hours or even several days, yet suddenly the family wants an impromptu discussion at odd hours. You do what you can, after all you went into medicine to help people, and sometimes helping means a lot more than diagnosing an illness, performing a procedure, or giving a medication.

Sometimes those family meetings were touching bonding moments, but still moments where the primary medical team should have bonded with a family, not some stranger (me).

For example, we were called to the ED to see and admit a diabetic patient. Yet, when we got there the patient was fine and could go home; except the family left the old lady there and refused to take her home until she ate something. The patient was in good health and had no reason to be admitted to the hospital and waste her time, our time and lots of medical resources. Our medicine consult was "patient won't eat." Some people not only have diabetic problems of high blood sugar (hyperglycemia) but also have low blood sugar (hypoglycemia), and some can fluctuate wildly between the two situations, often termed "brittle diabetes," because they seem to suddenly break one way or the other (too high or too low) very quickly and unpredictably. Evidently this lady had a hypoglycemic episode earlier in the day from not eating, so the family feared she would have another episode of hypoglycemia if she went home without an eating plan. Why did the ED need a medicine consult for this? The usual answer to everything in the ED is "We don't have time," everything in the ED is about time metrics.

In this harried ED environment, the medicine intern talks with the diabetic lady who does not eat. It was a pleasant bonding situation, one of those situations you cherish as a doctor, except you have about three other directions you are supposed to go while meeting with this patient. Turns out she would not eat, because no one gave her anything she liked to eat – does not take a doctorate level of education training to figure that out. In the ED, after they stabilized her by giving her some intravenous medication to increase her blood sugar (an Amp of D50: sugar solution injection), they gave her a peanut butter sandwich and basically said, "Here eat this." She said, "No," and the family said, "That's it, we're not taking her home like this." I talked to the elderly patient, who indicated she would not eat peanut butter (She did not like it, and it stuck to her dentures.) but would consider something else. Food pickings are slim in the ED late night, but she did agree to eat a ham sandwich (She preferred wheat bread, but we only had white bread). Mission accomplished, she could go home. Perhaps if we give older people good tasting food, many of these occurrences would be avoided.

In another sad situation, a person died and the family needed someone to talk to. I was only initially called there to write a death note. Again, another touching situation, which would have been better had my pager not kept going off. We talked, I listened a lot, they cried, we hugged. Again, the consoling stranger.

You never really knew who was going to have an urgent event, but it often seemed the patients the medical teams were most concerned about did fine and the ones in which no one suspected a problem suddenly had life-threatening issues. In the end, it is the lowly intern and a more senior resident bonding with the patient and patient's families at odd hours under strained circumstances.

Regarding society's ill falling on the ED doorstep, I was working ED rotation and met a young woman, her husband, and child on a very late Friday night. She was a cocaine addict ruining her life and destroying her family. She took a lot of drugs and her husband brought her to the ED. He was distraught, and their young daughter was sleepy. The patient told me, "it's like the Devil's got ahold of you", regarding her cocaine addiction. The husband stated he was through and either his wife gets rehabilitation for her drug problem or he is leaving, taking their daughter with him, and getting a divorce. Unfortunately, withdrawal from most drugs, other than alcohol and a couple others, is not a life-threatening emergency or a "medical condition." Hence, the argument was there was no "medical reason to keep her in the hospital." Of course, being Friday night, no social service rehabilitation programs would be available until Monday morning and most shelters were not keen on taking in active drug abusers if they could help it. What is the likelihood that this woman would slip back into her habit over the next two days? My guess is about 100%. Sadly, there was no way to get her admitted into the hospital. God and her family know what happened; I do not. I pray she got the help she and her family needed but fear that the most opportune time to help a drug addict is that moment they realize for themselves "I need and want help," may have passed.

A very sad story was a man with a stroke. I was not in Internship at that time, but on-call during physical medicine and rehabilitation residency year. All stroke patients are vasculopaths, meaning they all have proven vascular disease. As persons with vascular disease (usually atherosclerosis), anyone with a stroke can have a heart attack and vice versa. A large area of infarct and loss of blood flow oxygenation and nutrients can have a large area of tissue damage and death. Those dead and injured tissues are not as strong, resilient, durable or trustworthy as normal tissues and can have catastrophic failure within hours to about a week after an infarct event. In the stroke patient, it meant a sudden bleeding into the brain, an unresponsive patient, emergent CT, and emergent neurosurgical consult and unfortunately a terminal patient situation where nothing could be done, except to call family. Telling a 12-year-old boy he was "going to be the man of the house now," still brings tears to my eyes.

Chapter 19
Ancillary Support, or Lack Thereof, Especially when On-Call

Imaging often became a problem in trying to get things done in a timely manner.

Radiology is historically an understaffed field with relatively high wages. The shortage is becoming a major health care issue because radiology has moved from the background to the forefront of patient care upon arrival at a hospital, often going through a scanner right off triage, before ever seeing a doctor.

The radiology staffing issues, especially on weekends, meant the Radiology Department may not have check faxed orders for several hours, if at all. Orders were slow to process. Then when an old image was required for comparison, another several hours to several days were required to obtain the comparison films. We ordered a chest X-ray (CXR) at 9:30 a.m. After I called personally, someone shot the film at 1 p.m. By 1:30 p.m., the radiologist had seen the film, but needed a prior film for comparison to see if the findings were new. This patient could have ended up hospitalized another day simply to have two X-rays compared, and if there is a change, treatment will have been delayed in the interim, if no change, the patient's discharge delayed another day.

At 11 a.m., a STAT MRI was ordered for possible acute cord compression. We were waiting on MRI results at 3 p.m. for a medical emergency from 11 a.m.

In one Medicine Department Mortality and Morbidity (M&M) meeting, the case was of a spinal epidural abscess being missed. Why it was a Medicine service M&M is beyond me, as it was entirely a miss by the general radiologist on call and seen quite obviously and quickly by the neuroradiologist the following morning. The situation went something like this: Patient presented with symptoms of high-level spinal cord issues. The patient was appropriately evaluated by ED and medicine departments and even a neurology consult was scheduled. The appropriate spine MRI was ordered and the abscess was simply missed by the interpreting radiologist. At that particular hospital, the radiologists were not instructors but a privately contracted group to read studies, and while one or two of those contracted radiologists were quite helpful, some were pretty antagonistic toward residents. Even when the medical intern and more senior resident questioned the on-call radiologist about the issue of incongruity between imaging and physical exam and looking for clarification and guidance, the radiologist did not want to be bothered. Patient was admitted and neurology confirmed general medical exam findings. The next morning, the MRI expert/neuroradiologist of the radiology group called the medicine attending physician to report a spinal epidural abscess at the upper aspect of the images.

Well, in the M&M conference, some people started getting pretty terse toward the intern and the second-year resident for not overriding the attending radiologist and not directly calling a neurosurgeon in the late night for the case. As if! As if a lowly intern or even a slightly less lowly second-year medicine resident has the ability, power and backing to override a seasoned attending physician radiologist and wake up a neurosurgeon from sleep to say, "I don't like what I see in this patient and the radiologist does not want to be bothered with me." Yeah, that's gonna go far, far enough to get disciplinary action against the intern. Mutiny is frowned upon in medicine. This situation is just another example of the issue of unlimited responsibility and no authority pinning people into a corner. I did speak up in support of the residents in question, at risk of getting me labeled as a troublemaker.

Later, in training at another facility, I found out how good some of the other support staff, like EKG techs, were in my internship facility because during Internship we had round the clock access to EKG machines and EKG technologists, which was a luxury, not available at my next facility, a county hospital government–union run place. At the next place, you had to first find an EKG machine yourself, then do your own EKG, presumably while you were drawing your own labs, wheeling the patient down yourself for a chest X-ray (CXR) as there was little patient transport service available and the X-ray Department was as bad as getting an EKG technologist. Not that the government–union facility did not have EKG techs, but only from 8 a.m. to 5 p.m., which means they were actually available from about 9 a.m. to 3 p.m. and seldom showed up when called. No, this was not one of those VA facilities under investigation. Seriously, I called for an EKG tech at 9 a.m., for a patient on the stroke rehab unit with acute chest pain and no one showed. When I called back, the answer was "I got tied up for a couple minutes so assumed you did not want me anymore."

The term "union labor" does not inherently have to mean bad attitude service, but unfortunately, some take great advantage of the difficulty of getting rid of a lousy, even dangerous employee, due to union protections. The term "government facility" likewise is not required to be second-rate and inefficient. A major part of the problem is that at too many government-union facilities the employees are not hired by the department they will work in but from some sort of centralized human resource department more concerned about complying with government quota hiring statistics than actually getting the right person for the job or screening for underlying destructive personal behavioral characteristics that could damage a department or a whole institution. How would a person, essentially appointed to a department by an outsider, have any department loyalty or even the least concern about any specific department? While many people just want a paycheck, when you put as much time, effort, money and yourself into the healthcare industry, you desire and even expect some career satisfaction.

Even something as simple as opening the cafeteria at odd hours or maintaining longer hours to feed the overnight staff was impossible in that facility. That same facility claimed to be in compliance with American College of Graduate Medical Education (ACGME) guidelines of making food available to residents, by stating the vending machines in a remote basement area, which were typically devoid of food and snacks by 3 p.m., counted as "providing food for the resident physicians and overnight staff."

Chapter 20
Reaching a Breaking Point

In *Mein Kampf*, Adolph Hitler sings praises for those who just suffer in silence. I guess Mr. Hitler would not have liked me very well but would certainly be pleased with much of the education system and medical training paradigm. Although most leaders and administrators in America – nay, in the world – would not liken themselves to Adolph Hitler, those in positions of power who think abuses should largely be shouldered in silence by the victim, do share a philosophy in common with Mr. Hitler.

Of course, when work or training situations are unfair, abusive or overwhelming, hospital administrators and your immediate superiors often act like you are the only one with complaints or issues, which is exactly how situations such as molestations go unacknowledged and unchallenged for decades. Imagine someone accusing Mr. Sandusky of molesting a child in the 1990s; such a person would have been tarred and feathered, drawn and quartered, perhaps killed without explanation. No one would dare believe it. Remember, almost a decade or more, before Mr. Sandusky went to trial, a woman had already complained her son was sexually molested by Mr. Sandusky, and nothing was done, and a separate accusation of a shower impropriety with a minor was reported by the young graduate student coaching intern which was somewhat addressed internally, but no formal charges were filed. A former Penn State student affairs administrator got a rough time for challenging the culture of football first, image above all, and the secrecy structurally allowing such atrocities to occur. Anytime you have a system where a certain class in society or an institution is protected from the rules and consequences of breaking the rules, inequities will occur.

The point is that when an abuse occurs in an organization, there usually are several places along the way where complaints get systematically hidden, downplayed or ignored. For example, in our medical school, if a student was abused in his or her surgery rotation and wanted to complain (obviously not relying on a surgeon's recommendation letter for future career plans), the complaint eventually went to a surgeon in an academic capacity. If you were not satisfied with the department result, you were free to complain to the more general academic channels outside the given department, but eventually a complaint will reach those non-clinical academics, who are married or have some other close personal or social tie to the person who is the focus your complaint. Remember, those administrators have been acquainted with one another for many decades while students come and go on a four-year rotation, so ignoring an unpleasant history of which new persons are unaware is easy, and the cycle of abuse repeats itself. Obviously, your complaint about the Surgery Department to a dean who is the spouse of the Surgery Department director will get buried somewhere along the way, and you will be labeled the "troublemaker" for reporting abuse.

Many academic institutions have this very incestuous relationship, whereby anyone making a complaint against a perceived wrong done unto them is the "outsider" making trouble. The close relationship between school officials is not a conspiracy. When you have married people with very specialized highly regarded skill sets or someone who can generate a lot of business for your organization, you will inherently make accommodations to attract such a person or persons, those accommodations could be ensuring employment for a spouse at the organization. But the situation of spouses or close friends in an organization could become a conflict of interest if the personal and work issues cross paths placing close individuals at odds on an issue, which may compromise ethics.

Similarly, many of the publicized mass shootings of recent decades, despite the terribly inaccurate or downright misleading media coverage, have a common tie to a failed academic system where complaints reach administrators only to be hidden or ignored. However, when events literally "blow up" on the news airwaves, no one holds the school administrators accountable.

I was a nontraditional college student, medical student and medical resident, which means I was old enough to have experienced an America where people had civil rights and did not think constitutional rights and basic human rights needed be taken away because one was a student. I was also old enough and experienced enough to know my complaints would go nowhere but made the stand anyhow, because sometimes someone needs to rise and shout out the wrong, just because it is wrong, even if complaining will not change a thing. Sometimes you fight or speak out because it is the right thing to do, not because you can win. At least then such administrators cannot hide behind the comments, "We never knew," because, yes at least there is a record of my complaint proving they did know.

Below is an excerpt from a complaint I had during Internship. Nothing was really held back, because as much as I wanted to be a physician and care for people, things had gone too far:
(---),

I do not know if you realize it or if you care but you are killing me. I now get chest tightness and a couple days ago noticed a tremor while holding some papers.

Since I just went from Night Float to a new service I am evidently "technically" not Post-Call, yet Since going into work Sunday am at 7 (and not having people pick up pagers from me until 7:30 or 8am) I have got approximately 9 hours of sleep (not all in a row and none of it in the last 30 hours). My body is sick and weary. I know I am likely suffering from depression, but don't need Lexapro, just a good couple days off per month or so.

I do not know if you realize, but I will have worked every holiday in 2004 and been on call most of them. I have missed 3 weddings and spent my own Wedding Anniversary on call and post call.

Since the start of residency I have not had 2 consecutive days off. I mean talking real days off not that 24hours during Post-Call night Fri am until call again on Sat am. That is not a day off.

Today I reached a frustration point where I do not care to be again. Something needs to be done about the hours. It's not a problem working a lot of hours, but is a problem when working those hours going from 24-30 hour shifts then double back later that same night (like the all day Sun until Mon a.m., then back Mon night). It seems the worst combination of possible work hours has been given. I know about "hours restrictions" and how it impacts scheduling, but (---) has to decide if education or "coverage" is the goal of the residency program. The theory and approach to scheduling needs to be different than its present state.

Although all the paperwork says your days off might not be on the weekends, everyone seems to be trying to limit days off to only the weekend. I'd love 2 consecutive weekdays off this year, unfortunately it does not look possible, perhaps next year (2005 is almost here).

Counting being Post call at 7am Sunday morning until you start 6am or 7am Monday morning is not a worthwhile refreshing day off. I know the "24-hour" is a "day off" will occasionally happen, it seemed to happen a lot to get Night Float personnel on weekend coverage.

I am very disappointed with my decision to come here, I regret the day I decided to move (---) higher on my Rank list, I could kick myself, I spend more days wishing I was dead than being alive. I certainly would not at this point recommend anyone come here for residency. It is a shame because people at (---) are nice and good teachers, but all I think of is day to day survival. I try to hold my temper but am very frustrated and angry and bitter with a work schedule so miserable as I have had thus far.

Hopefully things can improve.

Jim

The reply:

Hey James,

Sounds like you need to request a vacation! Why don't you do that and I can give you a consecutive 7 (or even 9 days off if you are on an elective). You may feel a lot better if you take one. I am concerned about some of the sentiments that you

*express. Why don't we discuss this in person
rather than over email. I'm rounding with the Med
team this month but I should be available any
afternoon to meet with you. Just page me when
you have a chance.*

Thanks!

(---)

I overstepped boundaries putting the truth on the line. The program recommended I seek counseling (must be something wrong with the victim). I was more angry than depressed, but better play the game and I got counseling rather than fight the system and be destroyed.

A selective serotonin reuptake inhibitor (SSRI) medication was prescribed. One side effect of the SSRI was almost an aphasia symptom, like knowing the answer but not being able to say it, or knowing you should know something very common to you, but it keeps slipping from memory faster than you can say it. For me it was mostly apparent during a conference when the instructor was talking about malaria, and I could not for the life of me say the words I knew very well, Plasmodium Falciparum. No, those were not my first baby words, but interest in sharks and malaria go back a long way for me. Also, I felt the need to tell (scream to) all the potential candidates for residency, "Whatever you do, do not come here," but the words could not come out. Hence, I stopped taking the antidepressants prior to any exam, to avert any potential memory impairment at such a critical juncture. After a short while I stopped taking the medication. Later, a family medicine doctor told me he felt antidepressant medication should be automatically administered to all medical residents until they graduated, because residency is a depressive time and the sleep benefits of antidepressant medications may help more in a sleep-deprived person than even the antidepressant effects.

An example highlighting the bitter irony in medicine: We had a conference on the "more human aspect of medicine." As expected, most of the residents had other duties and could only attend a small portion of the conference.

The speaker was talking about compassion and passion in medicine and the perils of detachment. He also acknowledged a known fact (which no one has done anything about): Idealistic medical students eventually become emotionally detached physicians.

To me, the reason is obvious: How can a physician be compassionate when no one shows compassion to him or her? As a resident, you work more hours in two days than most people work all week, but you work those kinds of hours six to seven days a week. Then you get no overtime pay for those extra hours, so you are essentially a slave, under the guise of "training," yet you have no time to study. On top of that, you paid a couple hundred thousand dollars for this privilege, and have a malpractice target on your back. At least a couple of days a month, a resident physician (especially internship year) feels like killing himself or herself; on the better days, you just wish you were dead but don't fantasize much about it.

Detachment is the only way you can survive. Things get so overwhelming you either laugh at the insanity or want to kill yourself. Thus, detachment becomes a survival skill. Whenever you really go out on a limb to help a patient, get a special consult or procedure, file mounds of paperwork so they can keep their current medication when an insurer changes pharmaceutical contracts (called formularies) or sign for them to have time off to heal, you get burned.

During training, you develop skepticism that a patient even wants to get better; they just see doctors to build future disability claims, which would be fine if they had real disabilities. Some patients do have real disabilities and Worker's Compensation injuries, but because so many people exaggerate or even fake claims, the system is bogged down, and doctors have to search for the ulterior motive bringing the patient into the office. Thus again, you detach to protect yourself from getting hurt emotionally and legally. Thus, the doctor/patient relationship has turned into the patient versus doctor relationship. You must desensitize yourself. After spending multiple years being broke and overworked, many get bitter and lose compassion.

Chapter 21
Superstitions, or Anything
that Makes Call Better

As a resident, you can become superstitious. I never understood how baseball players could have superstitious activities to keep a hitting streak alive, until internship year. Then I was paranoid to shut off the lights in the call room, because once the last light goes off the pager comes alive. But getting comfortable sleep in a well-lit room is difficult. I would lie in bed trying to sleep, but constantly being awoken by the pager or lying in dread that the pager will go off any moment and feeling my pulse race and blood pressure pound in my ears. Eventually I gave up even trying to sleep. I have heard that a certain torture is to awaken a prisoner every hour. It seems like torture, yet for medical residents, especially Internship year, that is your life. Conclusion: Medical Life is Torture.

A friend relayed a story of a resident colleague who had his wife light a candle during his on-call nights. One night the guy was getting slammed, and he called home to ask if his wife had lit a candle. She indicated she had not lit a candle yet for his being on call. He half-scolding, half-pleading, stated, "Light a candle, light a candle!"

I had a lucky shirt, which seemed to result in fewer pages on a given night. The other superstition is that of having a full versus empty stomach. It's kind of a Murphy's Law thing: If you eat before work, you will have the chance to eat at work, but if you go to work hungry you will be so busy that you will not get a chance to eat. I remember going in one day, planning to do sign-out over dinner. Fate had a different plan – a code was called as I entered the hospital doors, and by the time everything was wrapped up, the cafeteria was closed. Then when midnight dining hours opened, I was again too busy to eat. I eventually developed the habit to always eat something before my shift started, and occasionally during shift, which only led to more calories.

You develop the bad habit of eating when you are not hungry, because a quick snack may need to carry you over skipped meals, but if you are already well-fed, then circumstances seem to allow that you can eat more, but if starving you get no meal. Thus, the fat get fatter and the starving starve. It's a viscous cycle.

Chapter 22
1-2-3 and We All Fall Down

Seems like every time I'm on call, someone, typically two to three patients, get confused and fall out of bed. In "House of God," the rule was called "Gomers go to Ground." Boy, is that true. For those not familiar with "House of God," the rather callous term "Gomer" stands for "Get Out of My Emergency Room." Generally, a gomer is a person for whom medical care is essentially futile; the patient has chronic issues not amenable to medical care, but since no one else can accommodate the person in their institution, the Gomer got sent to some hospital's emergency room. For example, some very elderly severely demented patients can be quite combative, which makes placing them in the appropriate care setting exceedingly difficult, because they can be a hazard to themselves, other patients and staff. Demented patients also wander, which has inherent problems, because if a demented patient is placed in a psychiatric wing and wanders into a paranoid schizophrenic's room, the consequences could be horrible due to a violent response by the startled schizophrenic. Delirium is like dementia but induced by illness or medication effects. You can imagine the outcome when a recent amputee patient forgets about the missing portion of a lower limb and steps out of bed onto nothing. People who do not have the strength to flinch their eyelids suddenly get the urge to get up out of bed to chase away imagined burglars, go to the bathroom (even though they have a catheter in), or feel like standing for no known reason. They seem to get those urges between about 10 p.m. and 6 a.m., God only knows why, perhaps. It is not right to just sedate everyone into next week. Having everyone constantly in restraint of all limbs (4-point restraint) is not ideal either, but letting people fall out of bed or wander incoherently around the building or city is no good. To make matters worse, laws have been passed to make safety features like a full bedside rail classified as a form of imprisonment. Waterboarding was legal, but having a full bedrail preventing someone from falling out of bed is bad. Hence, now all beds must have either incomplete rails or split rails so as not to be classified as prisons. Of course, that means purchasing all new beds; legislation forcing health institutions to spend more money is not a way to decrease healthcare costs.

These days, in response to patient falls and other issues, the government will not pay for any "hospital acquired" conditions, of which falls is one of the conditions listed. The law is an amendment to the 2007 Social Security Act, which gave CMS authority to implement payment changes to discourage hospital acquired conditions and required the Secretary of Health and Human services to identify at least two such hospital-acquired conditions to be addressed; 10 conditions are currently listed. Yet another example of back door implementation of a law having nothing directly to do with the original bill under consideration. In other examples, the healthcare legislation changed the student loan system, the reducing Americans vulnerability to ecstasy (RAVE) act was attached to the Amber alert child abduction legislation, credit card legislation resulted in a law allowing guns in federal parks and the troubled asses relief program (TARP) delivered a mental health parity and addiction equity act. TARP did not reinstate Glass-Steagall protections. The political beauty of riders is a politician can dissociate himself or herself from any undesirable legislation, by blaming someone else or the rider, yet use the rider system to personal and special interest advantage. I saw a "No Riders" bumper sticker when I was a child, but thought it was someone expressing opinion on hitchhiking.

The National Business Coalition on Health outlined the details of "Hospital-Acquired Condition Payment Policy" in the August 2009 publication healthcare purchaser tool kit. Hospital costs associated with a fall during a hospital admission will not be paid. Dr. Inouye et al. gave their impression of the consequences and unintended consequences of including falls as an element of hospital acquired conditions in the New England Journal of Medicine 360; 23 June 4, 2009. We hospital workers are told by administrators the government will null and void the entire bill for an entire hospital stay if a patient has a fall. Yes, spend a month in the ICU, a week on the medical floor, and have slight uninjured fall getting up from the toilet, and Medicare will refuse to pay for the entire hospitalization. Although the situation sounds like an exaggeration by hospital administration, the law inherently allows tremendous leeway for the government to determine how much of the cost is related to a patient's disease and how much of the cost is related to the "hospital acquired condition" and CMS decisions cannot be challenged.

In radiology residency we discussed the situation of catheter infections, because that is another hospital-acquired condition on the list. Sure, if you put a catheter access in a patient and two days later the patient has a catheter site infection, it is likely a catheter placement process-related infection, but what about the patient who has some infection at 30 days, the chemotherapy patient inherently prone to infection due to a compromised immune system, or the patient who already has an infection and you are placing the line to allow antibiotics to be efficiently administered? These are real issues facing physicians, department chairs and hospital administrators every day. I do not know how any business can survive under such a situation, and many do not. So rather than paying the legitimate hospital bill, the government re-writes its own bill where it may refuse to pay anything, or may be "generous" and pay a diminutive self determined portion of the costs. Financing the aforementioned situation is probably why I was recently charged over $560 for simple neck x-ray. Small wonder the hospital and other facilities under strong government regulation all get in line to beg, borrow and grab taxpayer funds to stay in business under the weight of not only unfunded mandates, but unpaid services.

Chapter 23
Everyone Wants Something

The rewards for "disability" can be significant in America, as potentially having a portion of your retirement benefits going untaxed is a huge incentive to "go out on disability" for many workers. The idea of "disability" seems to me to be for the truly disabled, and for the "work disabled" it should be work-related. All too often, relatively minor conditions, inconveniences or injuries that can heal in entirety are classified as "disabilities." My suspicion is that along with a usury tax system disability claims and worker comp claims also drive businesses away from U.S. shores, because as mentioned in a previous chapter, the wages in 2013 were at about 1979 levels in absolute terms for most industries and even lower when inflation adjusted. Since the Americans With Disabilities Act does not specify a list of allowable disabilities and the term "reasonable accommodations" is not defined, the terms "disability" and "reasonable" are as malleable and politicized as the terms "underserved area" and "underrepresented minority." Hence, although someone may think Parkinson's disease, cancer therapy effects, limb amputation, or spinal cord injuries are "disabilities," you may find that Carpal Tunnel Syndrome is the more common disability claim. While I understand that Carpal Tunnel Syndrome and back pains can be painful, they also seem to be an easily abused category for getting benefits.

I had a patient concerned about being denied a job due to a thyroid cancer diagnosis, which was treated and hopefully cured, time will tell. The people that manage such issues of discrimination based on a pre-existing medical condition at my institution agreed to help the person if needed and sent me a case example. The case example was a carpal tunnel syndrome claim, where it occurred to me the employer was very generous in giving the worker four different job opportunities to accommodate the person's real or feigned disability. The person chose one job position, but a few years later the company had a restructuring. The company made three options available, none acceptable to the employee, and so the employee sued under the Americans With Disabilities Act claiming the company did not make "reasonable accommodations." Under the act's vague terminology, the company lost. But America lost, too, because if you do not think that company or the next company will be looking to replace people with a computer or to take business overseas to avoid excessively liberal interpretations of Americans with Disability Acts rules, you are sadly mistaken.

Some of the tax breaks or government subsidies made sense in a prior era where the patient shouldered the cost of a disability himself or herself, but in an era where much disability burden is actually carried by the taxpayer, such extra tax exemption benefits are needlessly generous. For example, if you had to build your own ramp to the house out of your own pocket money, then the tax break for disability makes sense, but if you are going to submit the bill to the insurance company, be reimbursed by government, or charity, then others are paying your bill, so you do not need a tax break to cover the excess expenses due to illness.

Of course, the same situation happens in personal injury cases and medical malpractice cases, where the economic cost calculations completely ignore the fact the victim will be cared for by the taxpayers for the remainder of his life and calculates as if the injured person paid 100% of all costs out of pocket. Hence, people can scam one system and milk another.

The other issue is that many employers now exercise a point system, but unlike the NBA or NFL, getting points is bad. So, if you are late for work because a tree fell on your house during a severe storm (true story), you get points against you. Garner enough points and you can automatically be fired. This point system schematic is a way companies try to trim the budget or fire someone without facing discrimination accusations. Some employers draw a hard line on injury and illness: That point system means that if you try to work while ill but come in late or miss a day unexpectedly, you will accumulate points and get fired. Perhaps firing someone for a legitimate illness would be illegal (especially under the Americans With Disability Act) and it certainly adds insult to injury, but once your illness (like cancer chemotherapy side effects) is transferred into the sterile "point system," then you are fired for getting too many points, not fired for being a victim of illness. Nice trick. Hence, those companies utilizing a punitive point system also kill a good work ethic, because it is safer to just stay off work for a long time, rather than risk building up points. When many companies are so antagonistic towards their employees, one is not surprised people are looking for more ways to obtain compensation and have no loyalty.

The following year in physical medicine and rehabilitation training I learned that all patients whose estimated disability is under one year would automatically be denied, regardless of merit of the claim. Hence in cases where persons may have a legitimate short or intermediate term disability, patients and doctors are coerced into long-term disability situation.

Chapter 24
It is Easy to Get Sued

The case presented in this chapter had the plaintiff's side presented in a local newspaper.

I am glad to have learned a lot about medical malpractice on someone else's mistake and someone else's money but do admit being quite bitter over the entire situation.

I should not have even been on call that fateful day, because of already being post-call the day before, meaning I went into work, worked a 30-hour shift, went home, came in, and was on call again at least for the daytime. The resident scheduled to be on call was on a clinical rotation outside the hospital building so the call pager was handed to me. Carrying the pager in the daytime, meant you were often interrupted during rounds and if you acted in the patient's best interests, you often missed or ended up late to noon lectures, which got you disapproving glances and occasional condescending comments regarding your lack of professionalism. The point is, that even in the day time, carrying the call pager meant incessant interruptions to your learning experience and just made you a warm body slave to deal with any issue anywhere in the hospital.

Some of the usual interruptions occurred, many of which could be handled by phone. Then came that life-altering page, "We need you to come pronounce." That meant I was to go confirm a dead person was in fact dead, pronounce the dead person dead and document the death: "unresponsive, pulseless, breathless, no heart or lung sounds on auscultation." That was the routine, and medical interns had that unsavory task all too frequently thrust upon them, even in daytime, even in situations where the person was a private doctor's patient.

So, knowing the routine, I went to the room, and saw the patient. The nurses seemed troubled, and when I confirmed the person was dead, the nurses broke into tears. You have to understand that good nurses – not the ones who possess the "I just dispense pills" attitude, but real, caring nurses – get very attached to their patients. Thus, the tears were not a remarkable finding. I perused the chart gathering information to make myself aware of the fatal illness and then write the Death Note ("unresponsive, pulseless, breathless, no heart or lung sounds on auscultation" – now you know the routine). This was a patient who was in a persistent vegetative state for at least a couple years, who had a GI bleed, which was apparently stabilized and some electrolyte imbalance for which appropriate oral salt powder had been written. As the patient had Do Not Resuscitate orders, no code was called when she was dying.

So, I did the usual, confirm the death, log the report and call the coroner, then call the outside attending physician. Pretty standard stuff, case closed. Boy was I wrong. Just after getting off the phone putting the matter to rest, I get a tap on the shoulder to go to the nursing supervisor's office. I wondered, "What did I do now?" Then comes the question, "Could an injection of potassium chloride kill someone?" Well, since I think that is in the lethal injection concoction given to death row persons, "Yes it can, why?" The patient likely got potassium phosphate instead of potassium chloride, but close enough for medical catastrophe.

Time to make some quick phone calls back to persons I had previously notified to update on this new unexpected issue. During our first conversation, the outside private physician was very nice and indicated that he was not the usual physician caring for that patient but his partner was away at conference. Apparently when the lady had her gastrointestinal bleeding (GI bleed) episode at the nursing home, the patient's regular physician recommended comfort care and allow the patient in the vegetative state to die peacefully. Instead, the nursing home called an ambulance and had the person sent to the hospital. The work-up for GI bleeding can involve colonoscopy, which requires bowel preparation. Most of us have the usual loose stools and diarrhea from the preparation, and the mild loss of some charged ion salts (electrolytes) does not affect most people much. Yet, some people can have significant loss of electrolytes that need to be replaced. Essentially the same oral or intravenous medications are given to adjust the electrolyte issue, but at different concentrations and at different rates. For example, replacing electrolytes by IV can take several hours whereas a salt in a little fluid (strong solution) or a pill form can be immediately swallowed, and eventually the normal digestive process can slowly restore electrolyte balance to the body. If you give strong salt solutions very fast by intravenous push, you can have electrolyte, chemical and osmotic changes very suddenly, which can be devastating or even deadly.

In this patient, the bowel preparation, led to an electrolyte imbalance, which could be corrected by oral medications. Since this patient was in a persistent vegetative state, she could not simply sit up and swallow a pill; she could not even acknowledge her own existence (which is one of the checks prior to administering medications – correct medication, correct dose, correct route of administration and correct patient). All of those checks are designed for patient safety and accurate dispensation of medical care. Unfortunately, patients in certain conditions, like unconscious states and persistent vegetative states, cannot provide the supportive feedback to assist in providing with accurate care; the nurse-patient interaction is disrupted and something simple like, "Hey what is this medicine for?" cannot be discussed. In this tragedy of error, the outside attending physician appropriately wrote an order in the chart for an oral electrolyte replacement "packet of K-phos." However, the pharmacy did not have K-phos packets. Most places would have sent up a K-phos pill or capsule to be crushed or opened, respectively. Instead, the pharmacy sent up concentrated electrolyte solution to the floor. Many hospitals in this country had a moratorium against concentrated electrolyte solutions ever leaving the pharmacy and getting to a patient floor. Actually, even in this hospital that medication was supposed to be strictly limited to use in the ICU, by an ICU doctor. So how the medication escaped to a general medical floor in the first place is unknown to me and a sign of bad luck.

Another seemingly unrelated issue was waiting to collide with the first. Syringes can be the sort that just taper to insert into a rubber female receptacle connected to a line, like the receiver portion of a nasal-gastric (NG) tube, or can be a coarse pitch screw fitting like the sort going into an intravenous line (Luer lock). A long time before I was in medical school, and long before the young nurse was even in nursing school, someone in purchasing decided 10mL bulb syringes were absolutely unnecessary, as they were used much less frequently than the more standard 60mL bulb syringes, which got used for almost anything you could squirt 60 cc of fluid at. A cubic centimeter (CC) and a milliliter (mL) are the same amount and the terms are often used interchangeably. So, without a 10cc bulb syringe to measure the small amount of concentrated electrolyte solution, the young efficient nurse, trying to be as accurate and precise as possible, used the only available syringe, the standard 10 mL injection syringe.

In summary, a very concentrated solution of replacement potassium phosphate (K-phos) was now in an IV syringe in the patient's room.

Per coroner inquest statements and internal root cause analysis review, the nurse took the aforementioned medication into the room to give it to the patient via NG tube but just at that moment gets a message to immediately leave the room to take a phone call. In a sad irony, the distracting phone call is from the court-appointed guardian of the patient, as no family lived in this state nor had contact with the lady for several years. The nurse and guardian converse, nurse goes back into the room and gives the medication IV instead of via the feeding tube. Patient dies suddenly, and in comes the lowly intern to pronounce the death. This very ill patient could have also thrown a fatal blood clot due to her chronic immobility or had a heart attack or stroke, however, she died in close time proximity (apparently immediately) after the nurse gave the medication, and the nurse believes she killed the patient. I cannot deny the facts as laid out by the nurse's own statement.

After finding out the nurse's story from the nurse manager, I made phone calls back to the attending physician, and he called the legal guardian and family, which had to be awkward at best, since apparently the dead person's children were lawyers living elsewhere.

The more difficult call was to the coroner's office, because I wanted a truly objective coroner investigation. When an old person in a chronically ill state dies the coroner often will decline interest in the case, which usually makes sense – there's no need to do forensics and autopsy when you already have all the answers. I had to disclose there was possibility of a medical error, which biases the investigation from the start. Hence, the coroner investigation would inherently be biased against natural causes and skewed toward medical error or malfeasance.

Someone over at the coroner's office got more than a little suspicious, and an inquest was performed to investigate if this could have been an "angel of mercy" killing.

In defense of the nurse: earlier that day the same nurse and I worked together on an even older but much more alert patient who developed sudden chest pain, and we quickly got her issue addressed. The patient was rapidly assessed, stabilized and sent to the Cath Lab. The nurse went very well above and beyond to help that elderly lady get the best and quickest access to lifesaving medical care, so from her efforts to save another patient and her expressed frustration when the cardiologist was balking at my request to come ASAP, I doubt she would have been an "angel of mercy killer."

Although the hospital's lawyer thought it a bit extreme to investigate the situation as a murder instead of an accidental medical error, fate worked out well that the coroner investigated the mercy killing angle, because that weighed heavily in the nurse's and hospital's favor when the family members later accused the nurse and entire medical staff of "murdering" their mother in the local newspaper. When you are in litigation, you are often not allowed or at least strongly advised not to talk to anyone, especially the media, but unfortunately that need for silence until after the matter is legally settled allows you to be demonized in the public realm for quite a while for a crime you did not commit. Media pundits love to make a career hyping up accusations and doling out condemnation in the court of public opinion while the accused is not allowed to defend himself or herself. I would have talked anyhow, but the newspaper did not ever try to get hold of me, yet they lied and stated, "They could not be reached for comment." When all was complete, I contacted the same libelous newspaper journal to see if they wanted to print the truth (people were now free to talk), and I never heard back from them. So, no, the news is not about truth, it is about a story (fiction/rumor/propaganda and hype).

I learned about media manipulation again when one of my brothers who works for a police department described a murderer's arrest. We were watching the news together, and in the background was some SWAT/Fugitive Taskforce Team video clips. My brother indicated the film footage in the background was not from the recent arrest of the murderer but old footage of a drug bust – just more media grandstanding.

Early on, we all had to meet with the hospital's legal representatives regarding the case and give our answers to many questions of great detail. It seemed an exercise in minutia, but it made me aware how every syllable of every word had imperative significance. The scrutiny also made me uncomfortable that every breath I uttered could be manipulated to initiate a legal grievance and used against me in a court of law. Think how many things you say that could be twisted in any fashion to incriminate you. Heck, saying "Merry Christmas" can have the ACLU labeling you as a Christian oppressor of others' viewpoints.

There was a Root Cause Analysis meeting, which is a meeting to get to the root cause of a failure leading to a bad event and determine ways to avert such issues in the future. The problems could be quite mundane or be something as tragic as an unexpected patient death. The idea is to objectively come to conclusions to improve the process, not to point fingers. This meeting is where I found out that someone of no medical capacity at all made the decision to no longer have 10cc bulb syringes. It also led to some insight as to why when a packet of powdered K-Phos was ordered the pharmacy did not just send up a pill for the nurse to crush into solution but instead sent concentrated electrolyte solution to the floor. I also learned that our hospital was nursing staffed at the twenty-fifth percentile (essentially systematically somewhat understaffed and overworked). I hope most of those revelations led to improvement of patient care and better staffing at that institution, but I was only a lowly intern and would be leaving in a few months.

The scary thing about such meetings is that you are still not really free to talk openly. In theory, a Root Cause Analysis meeting is supposed to be a frank open discussion to have some good results and is supposed to be immune from prosecution and legal seizure/discovery. The reality is anything and everything can be legally seized and used against you. Silly emails from many years ago can and will be used against you. Yet, you cannot seem to get the emails that would possibly protect you – unless you are an IRS official targeting opposition political groups, then you can have unethical and possible criminal offenses suddenly disappear from a government computer and all the government computer backup storage, too.

I did not hear anything for quite a while, then suddenly received a legal document in the mail and was contacted by the hospital lawyer. He patiently explained things to me in great detail, and I was quite impressed. I mentioned that the lawyer sending the recent notice seemed like an imbecile making a bunch of nonsense statements and ludicrous allegations, yet I was always led to understand medical malpractice lawyers were pretty sharp individuals. The hospital's lawyer informed me there was a prominent malpractice attorney who took the case, bargained with the hospital for what seemed a reasonable settlement, but the family balked, wanting more. I do not know how much the actual money was and how much more you can get for a dead person who was in the condition of a potted plant while alive, but the family wanted more, allegedly very much more. Since the family rejected the settlement, the prominent malpractice attorney walked away from the case.

The second attorney was the probate lawyer for the will, and as I suspected he knew nothing about medical malpractice, except apparently cast a wide net and attempt to implicate everyone –the outpatient doctor, ER personnel, hospital staff, and even the lowly intern signing the death note. The guy was so bad, the hospital lawyers had to help him sue the hospital. For example, the plaintiff lawyer did not seem to understand that accusing the nurse of murder essentially released the hospital of malpractice obligations from the incident. He did not understand that a regular nurse he had used to sign off on the case is not qualified to evaluate a MD's medical decision (besides the fact that all the medical decisions were actually correct). Filing dates and proper structuring of paperwork would have been missed by the plaintiff attorney if not for the hospital attorneys coaching him. He eventually withdrew the case and got someone else to do it.

The actions of the third plaintiff lawyer is where I learned how sneaky and tricky the U.S. legal system can be against innocent defendants. Since the lawsuit took so long, I was done with Internship and elsewhere while the case was still pending. At one point, a notice was sent to my next employer (the previously mentioned government-union facility), and the legal department there never notified me. Fortunately, the attorney for my Internship hospital was on top of things (He warned me about the upcoming newspaper article accusing us of murdering an old lady.), told me of pending paperwork, and had filed our statement already. Good thing, because it turns out the paperwork sitting in the legal department of my government-union hospital contained a legal phrase indicating that failure to respond on my part indicated automatic guilt and automatic court case forfeit. Scary to think there's a time bomb clause making you automatically guilty of a crime you never committed or make you lose a civil suit you were erroneously named in the first place can occur in a nation that is supposed to pride itself on freedom and justice. Yes, in the United States if someone sues the wrong person and the defendant never actually gets the notice, a judgment can be automatically rendered against you as the defendant. Those days of having been served legal notice are apparently gone; you are now guilty until proven innocent, and if the plaintiff attorney intentionally or accidentally sends notice to where you are not, you lose. We are not as far from a Stalinist Soviet Union as some would have us believe. In my experience, we have now become much of what we in the United States used to say was wrong with our enemies.

The legal wrangling continued with the third plaintiff lawyer on the case and until I got some of the final paperwork, I did not realize that lawyer tried to accuse me of covering up a murder. So evidently facts and truth have no place in court. After much argument, that I never belonged on the lawsuit in the first place and after, thank God, the judge dismissed the murder cover-up allegations, I was finally removed from the case. There was even a Good Faith motion filed against the plaintiff attorney. A Good Faith motion actually means Lack of Good Faith equals tossing around unfounded accusations and making unfounded implications in a court of law. Unfortunately for me, apparently some of the ludicrous charges filed by the third plaintiff attorney, which ended up in the Good Faith motion filed on my behalf, was used as leverage for the hospital's settlement. Hence, I do not think I could sue the lawyer for his false accusations, because that option was allegedly used in the settlement. Long story short, a prosecutor or plaintiff attorney can make up all sorts of lies and is free to do so; you just have to pray the judge is not fooled by those lies. Hence, I propose there should be a two-year moratorium before prosecutors can run for a political office, because such a waiting period will give a chance for honest people railroaded by the legal system to raise objections and have the prosecutor's behavior examined, rather than have an abusive prosecutor ride the "tough on crime" mantra into a political career. I filed a complaint with the Ohio State Bar about such horrific life ruining behavior and overt lies by that attorney; the official statement was it was not their jurisdiction. When I replied stating how I found it implausible that such conduct of overt lying was acceptable to the State of Ohio Law Board, I was instructed the matter was closed, because they considered my good faith motion to have already addressed the issue. Since my good faith motion was evidently dropped as part of the settlement, I have no legal recourse and that lying lawyer faced no consequences for unethical behavior.

I have little faith in our legal system. It is a game where money wins, political favors are played out and egregious lies and deceitful exaggerations by prosecutors and plaintiffs are welcome.

Chapter 25
The Most Dangerous Time

The most dangerous time in a hospital was during nursing shift change. The nursing sign-out was sacrosanct and if you are inconvenienced, sick or dying during that time period, too bad.

Seriously, you would think some arrangement could be made to have nurse coverage at shift change time, but it seems nowhere I have worked had addressed the issue. This is many decades of patterned behavior, perhaps centuries of nursing tradition.

Yes, the medication schedule of diabetic patients needed to be changed to allow for nursing shift change sign-out, and nursing sign-out apparently must take place away from anywhere they could possibly be disturbed.

Pray you do not have a heart attack at sign-out/ shift change, because you will be unattended. Sure, your doctor would still help you, but unless the doctor coincidently stumbles across your peril you will be suffering awhile, because there will be no nurse to call the doctor.

I do not know how something so detrimental even potentially deadly, to patient care has survived as routine practice for so long. I guess it is because nurses have unions and doctors don't. I suspect as the healthcare system obliterates the doctor-patient relationship and drives all doctors into subservience employment, then doctors too will become the worker drones of Karl Marx's alienation of labor philosophy and then the doctors too will unionize, stop in the middle of anything for break time and stop practicing at 5 p.m., even if it means stopping chest compressions or surgery.

The only thing more detrimental than the sanctity of nursing sign out is a passive-aggressive angry nurse who leaves out important patient care information at sign out or who forgets to tell the oncoming nurse about medications the current nurse was supposed to give patients, but did not get around to administering. Otherwise, the new nurse expects the patient has already been treated to date and all previous shift orders were performed. This was especially an issue with paper charts, where once a medication list was turned to a new page it was evidently against all laws of reason to ever turn back one page and make sure everything was indeed done. I do not know if computers will help, as being too lazy to scroll down the page or click to another window to assure medications were given will have the same problem, just at greater infrastructure expense. The days of reprimanding a bad nurse have gone, it is usually the person making the complaint who is punished. Such a situation makes the work environment frustrating for the good nurses who must pick up the slack and dare not complain. Some of those great nurses, get tired of the situation and bureaucratic burdens and go into medical management or leave healthcare altogether.

Chapter 26
Comedy of Errors Code

I remember one of my first codes. A "code" in a hospital means a certain issue has happened and requires an immediate response. When doctors talk of "codes" we usually mean someone had suddenly passed out of consciousness, whereby breathing and heart support may be required urgently. We call it cardiac arrest if a heart attack (aka myocardial infarction, infarct of the heart muscle [although nerve tracts in the heart can be damaged too]) and call it pulmonary arrest of the person stops breathing. Cardiopulmonary arrest if both heart and breathing stop: Such a patient needs resuscitation to survive, keep blood perfusion, and get some airflow into the lungs. Keeping blood flow is the top priority, so chest compressions in CPR (cardiopulmonary resuscitation) is absolutely necessary, with establishing airway ventilation following close behind. Other situations happen where a patient is so out of consciousness that even though the patient is breathing and has a heartbeat, such a patient may not be able to protect his or her airway. Such a patient cannot swallow normal secretions from the mouth glands and cannot gag if something "goes down the wrong pipe," so to speak. In such a patient where secretions and/or contaminates or vomit can enter the airway and even the lungs, the outcome could be asphyxiation, but more often aspiration pneumonia, a life-threatening lung infection, occurs.

Such an aspiration pneumonia occurred to a patient I met in the ICU. The woman had undergone gynecologic (GYN) surgery and had some post-operative bleeding. The chief OB/GYN resident got the clever idea of just placing the patient in Trendelenburg position (the head is below the level of the body and feet). The patient was drowsy after operative anesthesia and could not protect her airway. The situation only gets worse when you leave such a patient in a head down position, with an unprotected airway indefinitely. The patient allegedly aspirated some stomach acid, which caused inflammation to the lungs and the patient got a trip to the ICU. Long story short, do not turn someone on their head to stop the bleeding, tamponade (put pressure on, Band-Aid) or suture/cauterize the bleeding site.

So, now you know a little about codes and airway protection, I will tell you a little about red tape.

Some people have a breathing condition where when they sleep they stop breathing for a while; it is called sleep apnea. For some people, the cause is neurologic, but for many it is obstructive in nature. For some people while sleeping on the back, the relaxed tongue falls toward the back of the throat and restricts airflow. Such a person stops breathing for a few moments, then usually has some sort of lurching to a mild or even severe degree, perhaps a snort, the tongue moves and the person breaths again. The process repeats itself all night. Snoring in such individuals is common, but snoring is not apnea, because the person is breathing regularly. Snoring is annoying to the spouse of such a person. The apnea is troubling to the spouse, because they notice their loved one repeatedly stops breathing. The only thing the apnea patient knows is that even after a long night sleep, he or she never seems well rested.

A treatment for obstructive sort of sleep apnea is a device to pressurize the airway: continuous positive airway pressure (CPAP). A CPAP is commonly used at home and you do not need an engineering, nursing or medical degree to use it. Yet, in the hospital a CPAP is a "respiratory device," which has a whole host of implications regarding nursing care, unit placement and bureaucratic red tape. Hence, some simple to use at home every day device becomes a bureaucratic quagmire in a hospital situation. So, yes, a guy with simple obstructive sleep apnea on the hospital overnight for a low-risk procedure or some issue not related directly to his breathing can lead to staffing battles, transfers to extraordinary levels of care and involvement of top administrative and ethics advisors. Don't even get me started about the insulin pump.

Within this background was a patient who had a code situation. Code Blue was the call for CPR. Most the code duties were run by medical residents and could be pretty intimidating if you were inexperienced, and the first person to the code was to take the lead. Some residents craved the opportunity to run a code, others dreaded it, a few may have avoided it.

The patient went into tachycardia (fast heart beat arrhythmia) and felt very sick, and if he changed from a tachy (fast) rhythm into a fibrillation (irregular rhythm that does not pump blood) he could die. Things looked bad. Also, the guy had a Do Not Intubate order, which means the usual medication, intubation, resuscitation and ICU transfer were not in the works. He also did not want to go through chest compressions or being shocked (defibrillated back to life). This was like a "do this with your hand's tied behind your back and blindfolded" sort of situation. Medical (medicinal) management was acceptable but no interventions. During this situation, the patient was very uncomfortable and just wanted the fan blowing fresh air on him, or at least the comfort of blowing air while he was in an impending dire situation. I held the patient's hand and spoke calmly with him. The person running the code kept stepping in front of the fan, which irritated the dying patient. Then every time the resident running the code mentioned what he wanted to do, there seemed to be some resistance to his orders. "Start an IV," to which someone answered, "I cannot get IV access," which led the resident running the code to state in exasperation, "Oh my God, this guy's gonna die!" The patient would then respond, "I'm going to die?" To which the code leader would reply, "No sir, you are going to be fine." And this cycle would repeat itself after each order was for some physical or policy reason unable to be carried out. "Give him (…) medication." "We don't have that on the crash cart." Oh, my God he's gonna die!" "I'm gonna die?" "No sir, you're going to be fine." As if it could not get more frustrating, when the discussions regarding whether the CPAP device represented intubation or not began, things entered the realm of the ludicrous. CPAP does not even use a tube and non-terminally ill people routinely use it at home, but was now on the verge of being considered extraordinary measure or not.

Eventually, we got some medication in him, which took effect, and he improved symptomatically. Still, he was at risk of imminent death. He knew he was seriously ill and going to die any time, just when and how?

Because he did end up with the CPAP machine, he was transferred to the ICU. His family joined him. Later that night, while I was on call, I heard the patient's monitor go very slowly, then stop, then a continuous beep, then nothing. A voice from the patient's room asked nervously, "Sir, what does this mean, is he dead?" as she pointed to the monitor with the flat line indicating no detectable heart electrical activity. I said, "Yes." He brady'd down and died. It seems when someone goes into a bradycardia (very slow heart rate), the process of death is more peaceful than with a tachycardia condition. Tachycardia conditions have so much more symptoms and drama associated with them, maybe that is because the struggle for life is still going, whereas bradycardia is like the switch is turned off and you power down into the hereafter.

I did end up taking the lead on a code quite by virtue of being in the right place at the right time, or the wrong place at the wrong time, depending on how you look at it. My senior resident and I were called to electively intubate a patient in a surgical intensive care bed. My senior got called to the ED, so I figured I would wait until he got back. Fate had different plans. Turns out the very person we were going to electively intubate suddenly coded, his heart slowed and stopped. It is easy to guess who was the first person in the room, already with intubation kit. So, here I was, first few days new resident running the code and intubating the patient. All I can tell you is that when things get too rough and the pressure too much, just go back to the basics, keep it simple. We successfully resuscitated him. Sometimes you win. Unfortunately, for all the medication paradigms, scientific studies and other procedures, the fact remains that a third of the time a person codes, they live; two/thirds they die, you can only do your best.

Chapter 27
Wilting Away

A 92-year-old person was admitted to the hospital and started on an aspirin (abbreviated ASA) 81mg p.o. daily. That particular dose is the cardioprotective dose recommended by the Bayer Corporation and cardiologists the world over. I would say once someone reaches 92 the treatment to promote longevity has already proven successful and now the risks may outweigh the benefit, especially in a person with history of stomach surgery (partial gastrectomy) for stomach ulcers. Another thing done is to give old people with loss of appetite, stimulants like Megace (progesterone analog) to increase appetite. Unfortunately, increasing appetite in someone too debilitated to feed herself or intolerant of food in the GI tract (causing pain, nausea and vomiting, with possible aspiration of food contents into the lung and subsequent aspiration pneumonia) could become an unintentional torture.

We worry when old people do not eat or when the memory fades. I do not know if such situations are a blessing or curse for the patient, but it is distressful to family members and medical care providers. Perhaps the body knows what it is doing. The natural course will be to one day shut down. Just as deciduous trees have internal programming to lose leaves before winter, we to have internal programming of aging, defined in DNA as the shortening of telomeres. None of us are getting out of this world alive. Think of the plant that begins an early bloom, only to get smashed by a late winter storm, it often fares worse than the plants that have remained without leaves until later in the season. Similarly, at some point it may be more harmful to interfere too much with the natural course of aging and dying. We need to grasp reality – we will age and die, if all goes well. At one point, medicine focused on stopping death, which made sense, because it was a win or lose battle. Now medicine can end in a situation, where the person is not fully alive, yet not dead either, but held in mechanically assisted limbo.

It's our natural decay - we decline, we lose appetite in harmony with our inability to obtain or tolerate food, we drink less water and our thirst drive is suppressed, our mind gets a little more loose and tangential in thought, as we are ready to pass from this world to another realm. We then get weak, tired, sleepy, cast off this garment of who we are (or think we are) and pass into the world beyond. If we interfere in the wrong way, we make death a most distressing experience. We all want to avoid death, even though we know it to be an inevitable part of life. *Maybuhay* is Tagalog word meaning, to live well. We cannot guarantee how long we will live, but we can do our best to decide how well we live.

Not to suggest that medicine should do nothing to avert untimely death, but perhaps medicine should not disrupt the natural passage out of this life too much. Life is distressing enough; we do not need to make death distressing, too. For instance, really consider what is to be gained by placing a demented person with a swallowing disorder on a feeding tube. Or placing a feeding tube in an old person who is fully cognizant but does not wish to eat and knows she is near death and welcomes it as salvation from the pains of living. Like many situations, one must ask, what is to be gained for the patient.

I am not suggesting euthanasia. I am against physician assisted suicide and do not suggest people die due to treatable depression. I'm simply suggesting that we live in harmony with our bodies and that medicine and society spend more effort on improving the quality of life than the quantity. Many medical professionals and insurance providers use death as the end marker of treatment efficacy and discount the value of treatments improving quality of life without change in mortality. I would rather spend a dozen of my last days on vacation than in the hospital for the same lifespan. I may even prefer a week of vacation on my last days rather than spend an extra month of life bouncing around various hospital units. I think hospice for terminal patients is along the lines of trying to make a smoother transition from life as we know it to whatever is next.

Chapter 28
Diabetes

Similar to instances of CPAP machines, I have seen the same bureaucratic battles happen from an implanted insulin pump. Some patients with diabetes are best controlled with an insulin pump rather than subcutaneous insulin injections at certain fixed time intervals and adjusted according to meal carbohydrate (carbs, sugar) intake. The device holds insulin and often has a catheter inserted into the patient, like in a thigh vein. The pump can be refilled as needed, and the insulin can be metered out in very precise doses. Once the team managing a patient's diabetes gets such an apparatus set it often works quite well and does not need a rocket scientist to use it. I remember a patient whom we had a terrible time controlling blood sugars, and I've learned a couple things from other diabetic patients as well. One thing I learned is that Qhs (standing for "in the evening") means something different in hospital time than outpatient time. For example, a patient who takes a scheduled insulin dose at Qhs often takes the does before bed-time, which in practical terms translates to approximately around 7 p.m. to 9 p.m. and tends to follow a fairly fixed schedule (like 8 p.m. every night, forever). In the hospital, I learned Qhs means in the evening and is interpreted as about 5 p.m. Hence, a diabetic person entering a hospital for any reason may inadvertently have their insulin schedule disrupted by two to four hours, and changed with respect to meals, which is a very significant impact on blood sugar management and can leave professionally managed hospital patients with worse blood sugar control than they can do on their own at home.

Another thing I learned from an ophthalmologist who was also a diabetes patient was that there is no such thing as a "diabetic diet," according to the American Diabetes Association (ADA). The ADA simply recommends covering carbohydrate ingestion with an appropriate amount of insulin. Yet, every hospital I have worked has a "diabetic diet." I found from discussion with nutrition staff that all a diabetic diet means is that the patient does not get a doughnut, muffin or Danish pastry for dessert. Seriously, pancakes with syrup and fruit juice to wash it down and mashed potatoes slathered in gravy are all OK for a typical hospital "diabetic diet."

My patient with the insulin pump was blind and lived with a couple of family members; none had more than a high school education but made a well-functioning family unit and managed the insulin pump just fine. Unfortunately, in the stroke rehab unit an insulin pump was like a NASA Mars unit and more dreaded than dismantling a nuclear warhead, hence absolutely forbidden due to nursing policy. Yes, that situation meant very skilled, well-trained nurses, therapists and doctors could not manage a simple device, with instructions already spelled out, that much lesser educated persons could manage at home without any issue. My dad considers that situation to be representative of trading in common sense for an education.

So, time to play the "chase the blood sugar game" with this patient. After much effort, consults with endocrinologist blood sugar experts and fruitless attempted medication adjustments, we asked the patient, "Why are we having such a problem with controlling your blood sugar? Even without the insulin pump you state you have few problems at home." We probably should have proactively asked the patient, "How can we best keep your blood sugar under control – what works for you at home?" His answer was straightforward and brief: "You are feeding me too much." We then looked back at his "diabetic diet" meals actually being delivered. Not even mentioning all the carbohydrate (carb)/sugar loading being done, we noticed he was getting the equivalent of at least two full meals at every meal. For example, one meal was a huge plate of macaroni and cheese while also including large helpings of roast beef with huge amounts of mashed potatoes and gravy along with the usual juices and breads (but no dessert pastry). He was getting unlimited calories and many of those were carbohydrate calories, so of course his blood glucose was all over the place. We adjusted his intake to limit total calories to a reasonable generous human calorie intake and his blood sugar was fine thereafter, even without the insulin pump.

Since I have mentioned diabetes, I will give my opinion, and that opinion is we have it partially wrong. We have about three ways to classify diabetes: Child onset versus adult onset; Type I versus Type II; and insulin dependent (insulin lacking) versus insulin resistance. The problem is there is erroneous exclusion criteria and overlap in some of the categories. For example, a typical Type I diabetic patient is a child who develops blood glucose issues after a viral illness of unknown identity. But how do you classify an obese child who gets blood sugar issues from similar clinical setting? Historically, all adult onset diabetes was called Type II diabetes but implies obesity-related and does not explain the thin adult with diabetes who had the same prodrome of viral illness prior to diabetes as a child did. Those classifications also do not explain why sometimes a person with Type II Adult onset diabetes one day needs insulin and the oral medications no longer work. I think the best way to classify diabetes is whether the patient is not making enough insulin versus if the patient is making insulin, but the body does not respond properly to the insulin present. Although many researchers recognize this concept of using insulin production versus insulin resistance to classify diabetes, in clinical practice measuring both insulin and blood glucose (sugar) levels is rarely done. Admittedly, glucose testing is quicker and easier than insulin testing, but for some patients the insulin level would help more precisely classify the type of diabetes and provide more appropriate management sooner. Yet people still get classified under the old vague categories, even in an era where we can have actual measurements. The current diabetes treatment paradigm is as follows: If you are trying one method of treatment based upon guesswork, but it is working, don't bother to ask questions. Such willful ignorance leads to situations where doctors and patients think they "have failed" when a diabetic treatment no longer works rather than acknowledging the physiology has changed or the wrong assumptions about the pathophysiology was made due to incomplete information. Such a situation of perceived "treatment failure" is frustrating to physicians and emotionally devastating to patients.

Part 5:

The Philosophical, Medicolegal-Psychosocial-Regulatory Practice Environment

Chapter 29
Nurse Practitioner (NP) and Physician Assistant (PA) Impact on Medicine as a Career

Nurse Practitioners are like a Master's or Ph.D. in nursing, which means they may be a "Nurse Doctor" who are not actual medical doctors but sometimes introduce themselves as a "doctor," as if that is not confusing enough for anyone, let alone patients seeking to see a medical doctor but end up seeing a nurse doctor or a doctorate of something else. Physician Assistants are supposed to be just that, *assistants.* I suppose we will have doctorate of sanitation, doctorate of cab driving, and secretarial doctorates, too? Where does this degree madness end? Politicians push for the never-ending degree climb under the pretense that higher degrees mean better service skills, and obviously it generates more income for colleges as people are coerced into higher degrees to keep their jobs. Seriously, you do not need a Master's or Ph.D. to teach fourth-grade history, you do need at least a fifth or sixth grade level history to stay ahead of the fourth graders. My example is a little extreme in that obviously we prefer adults running a fourth-grade classroom, and teachers should have some education above high school, but the point is many skills required in being a good teacher, like good communication of the topic knowledge to children, not attacking or molesting children are more important characteristics than degree level. I do not know that a "Master's in Music" person teaches music any better or plays the piano any better than when he or she was a teacher with a Bachelor's degree. In fact, the extra time spent working on higher degrees may be a diversion from actually teaching and refining his or her music talent.

There has been such big use in the services of Nurse Practitioners and Physician assistants and now even many Physical Therapists and Occupational Therapists have advanced degrees, that there is no longer a reference to "your physician;" we are all now "providers." In fact, many places do not even refer to patients as "patients" but as "clients," Why is this important? It is important, because the Hippocratic Oath never referred to a "Provider-Client" relationship; the Hippocratic Oath was between a Physician and Patient. Thus, the very foundation of the medical relationship has been destroyed. Sure, most physicians try to keep the relationship, but under the "Provider-Client" healthcare system, it is impossible to provide the relationship expressed and implied by the Hippocratic Oath, no matter how hard you try.

Some of the problem is that as reimbursement for seeing any individual patient became lower, doctors have to run patients through like cattle, and as compliance and billing gets more technical it takes more hands and eyes to keep out of trouble and get paid, hence utilization of PA and NP services. We called this "Managed Care." Under managed care, you could be stuck with a doctor you did not personally mesh with, or you felt was rude or incompetent. Under the more free market fee for service system prior to managed care, people would eventually stop seeing such a physician and that physician would have to change for the better or do something else. Since people could not leave an unsatisfactory medical relationship under the managed care model, people yelled to the same politicians who helped create the mismanaged managed care system and hollered to the media, with a resultant myriad of oppressive regulations and more levied on medical students and doctors. Unfortunately, some doctors were also lazy, or became lazy, and let these other "providers" essentially take over many "doctoring tasks", until these providers now demand the same privileges as physicians and many politicians grant them those privileges. Again, this makes a further disconnect between physician and patient.

I think the greatest coup was for politicians and media to convince people the government was the good guys and doctors were evil. Doctors take an oath to heal and help people and those are the "bad guys" while politicians trade influence for money – and they are the "good guys"?

PA's lobbied politicians essentially saying, "There is a shortage of doctors in 'underserved" areas gives us the authority to do it." Of course, like all political promises, these were broken and the majority of PA's, NP's and other "providers" still practice in the major cities or large suburbs, and the "underserved" are still underserved.

Now do understand, "underserved" in America is a political entity, just like the "underrepresented minority," and the definition can vary with the political winds. For example, the same "underserved area/underserved population" for getting taxpayer money funneled to your hospital for a building project or to expedite a foreign doctor's VISA application is not necessarily "underserved" for getting an American citizen and American-trained doctor some government credit or tax deduction regarding his or her student loans.

The term "underserved" is a political moving target and often leaves a population over-served in things they do not want or do not need and lacking in areas of true need. Hence, I know of general hospitals that are much better equipped in caring for cancer patients than some cancer specialty hospitals. In fact, in places like Buffalo, N.Y., even dedicated cancer, heart and neurologic facilities were about a decade or more behind good community hospitals in Michigan regarding up-to-date standard of care (not to mention "state of the art" care often more available at good community hospitals in other states). Of course, New York is a state with strong government influence. When I say "government influence," think of the idea that your money is not your money, but your right to pay high taxes – think of that communist "command economy" model again – and you understand why many places in New York are so far behind. From my experience, the more government affiliation such institutions have, the farther behind in standard of care they seem to be.

Much political finagling and perhaps some laziness on the part of doctors has now given NP's and PA's almost as much privilege as doctors at about a tenth the financial cost of obtaining a medicine education, less actual classroom and on the job training experience, not to mention the cost of life efforts (PA's and NP's do not work 30-plus hour shifts and over 100-hourworkweeks at no overtime pay.) At the end of the day, when the cliché "Shit hits the fan" and "The going gets tough," it is "Doctor, Doctor, call the Doctor!" The physician has ultimate responsibility but little authority these days. Of course, when lawsuits happen, lawyers are searching for names of "doctors" to place in a lawsuit, not the other "providers." Some lawyers have cast a pretty wide net (as indicated in chapter 24) but suffice it to say, malpractice money is made in suing doctors and hospitals. Now, although celebrities can apparently give medical advice, essentially "playing doctor without a license" like telling women not to get the appropriate radiation therapy concordant with lumpectomy for certain breast cancers, such persons are not held responsible for their potentially deadly misinformation. Ultimately, when people get drugs from a dealer on the street or take medical advice from celebrities, if something goes wrong they sue the doctor, not the street drug dealer or the celebrity. I even remember a TV commercial where the person actually stated, "I'm not a doctor, but I play one on TV"; evidently it had advertising credibility better than a real doctor.

With every nurse, physician assistant, nurse practitioner, therapist, various assistants and other "providers" taking a portion of what was once a general practice/primary care doctor's domain, there is not much left for a general doctor to earn a living from. Also, since the PA, NP, therapist and every technologist training route is much cheaper and starts paying a salary much earlier than full medical training, the economics of such competition and long delayed financial compensation weigh against many potential physicians being able to afford to go into the primary care specialties.

Yes, almost all nurses make more money than a medical resident, yet when a patient's life is on the line in the middle of the night, it is the lowly resident who is ultimately called and responsible to save the person, not the other "providers."

Obviously if the answer is, "It no longer makes economic sense to become a general practice physician under the current U.S. healthcare model," then either something has to be done to make primary care more appealing (scholarships, better salary, less regulations, litigation protections etc.) or we must accept the fact that physicians will be driven into specialty practices to get said protections and compensation. The protections come from less competition from non-physician personnel and limited practice scope, which means limited litigation scope and limited billing scope. The limited billing scope means lower billing and coding service costs and less chances for a billing mistake getting you unpaid or labeled a criminal.

The point is that while judicious use of ancillary support staff can result in efficiencies, the overuse of such services can be confusing and detrimental to the entire structure of the healthcare system – and the outcome likely already has been deadly to patients.

Not just doctors, the nursing paradigm has also changed. Prior to the 1990s, an RN was good enough for nursing and nurses provided direct care for patients, but in the 1990s there was a strong push towards requiring all nurses to obtain a Bachelor of Science in Nursing (BSN), in no small part to justify a relatively high salary for someone not having a full college degree. It seems to me people with a full college degree are going to be averse to changing bedpans and diapers, compared to someone who just wants to take care of patients. I remember overhearing a conversation between a couple of nurses while I was in medical school. A nurse's assistant of some classification was cleaning a bed because a patient had a very messy diarrhea episode, and the nurse would not help. I overheard the nurse stating, "I have a degree and dispense medications." In fact, that same nurse would not even get a different patient a drink of water, because that was not her job and stated to another nurse the patient would get a drink of water when the assistant cleaning up the diarrhea patient's room was available. Few younger nurses seemed satisfied in patient care, and many I met were maneuvering into other avenues. BSN's were going on for Nurse Practitioner degrees, RN's were working on BSN degrees, and LPNs were working on RN degrees, which means a lot of nurses were not settled into where they wanted to be. Nurses' aides are used a lot, which can be a great help in "assisting" with patient care, but dangerous when they become the "replacement" for hiring appropriate nursing care. When a nurse's aide documents horribly low or high blood pressure, or ludicrously high or low blood sugar on an unconscious patient, it means nothing to that assistant; it is just a number. Well, those numbers actually mean something and could mean something critical, but just get written down onto a paper or entered into a computer, left to sit until an actual nurse or doctor stumbles across the serious information to address the situation. For example, while I was in Physical Medicine and Rehabilitation (PM&R) residency, one of the residents was expressing frustration of finding out a patient had been unconscious and had a ridiculously high blood pressure, high enough to cause a stroke, and no one reported the values to a physician to address this deadly issue. Hence, all these classifications and re-classifications of healthcare "providers" to modify the budget is not good for patient care, because the nurses are distracted from the role of nursing, and nursing aids are overwhelmed by duties no one else wants to do and expectations they are not trained to manage.

In a paradox created in part because many non-physician hospital employees have union representation leading to education benefits and more flexible work hours, it is not unusual for nurses, therapists and social workers to have business management degrees at least partially sponsored by their employer, which sets up a situation where eventually the social workers become the bosses or entrepreneurs and the doctors are essentially assembly line employees. Hence, the preferential ability for non-physicians to attend graduate business and healthcare policy sorts of programs is just another way physicians are minimized in the healthcare equation.

Finally, while the appropriate use of ancillary support staff, including mid-level providers, may have some profitability in a business model, the current medical reimbursement system actually punishes efficiency. The thought is similar to the Joe Biden philosophy of "You did not build that." Hence, your efficiencies in providing medical care belong to the government, not you. Therefore, your efficiencies do not mean more money to your medical practice institution, but mean the government and private insurers get to pay you less for your services. In the long run, you work longer and harder to keep the same pay while the next generation of physicians and other healthcare workers face escalating expenses and lower wages. A sign at a warehouse I once worked stated: "The beatings will continue until morale improves."

In summary, while certain benefits to patients and certain efficiencies can be obtained by having additional "providers," the roles of various providers in the healthcare system need to be clearly defined and utilized appropriately. Also, there needs to be a system to stop punishing physicians and organizations for efficiencies and improvement in patient care.

Chapter 30
Priorities

In medicine, we should and do rightly focus on what we may consider untimely deaths. Most of those untimely deaths are better served by prevention than medical treatment, but the old adage that an ounce of prevention is worth a pound of cure has seemed to be forgotten in present society. Avoiding an accident is better than going to the emergency room after one. Best to stop smoking than requiring physicians to place you on a respirator to help you breathe. Better to watch your diet and weight than require CPR. Challenge one in a boxing ring, on the tennis court or on a soccer field rather than shoot someone with a gun. Perhaps one day all battles of war can be decided by Academic Challenge, martial arts or a team soccer victory.

We know the horrors of violence, but what of the horror of smoking or other vices? Smoking and driving under the influence of drugs and alcohol all kill many more people than terrorism in yet the United States (along with many other nations) spend billions to trillions of taxpayer dollars on not only fighting actual terrorism overseas, but on fighting perceived terrorism, while spending comparatively little regarding the things taking the most lives. Yes, US drone program kills people without any due process, probable cause, trial or jury and if you think such a killing paradigm inherently excludes you and your family, you are delusional. For a nation like America, freedom and due process are imperatives to our national definition. Not that a government should ignore security threats, but prioritizing the amount of taxpayer funds on addressing a given threat be in some way proportional to the actual statistics, not to media-hyped emotional aspects.

Just as disproportionate priorities and disproportionate responses can be devastating for society, they can harm the body as well. The media incessantly projects an edited propagandized viewpoint of man's inhumanity to man in graphic detail, but the tragedy of vices fall silently by the wayside. There is no daily blaring imagery of people with wrinkled faces, yellow and missing teeth wheezing for breath with their oxygen masks every night on the news. Perhaps when small pox and the plague devastated the earth smoking risk was easily ignored, but now since most people in developed countries do not die of famine and disease in childhood and infancy, the impact of smoking is much greater in cause of death statistics and needs to be addressed in the media, not just the intensive care unit, hospice, and cemetery. Only the occasional shock tragedy is shown and then quite briefly. Thus, the victims of self-destruction by reckless driving, drugs, alcohol, smoking, sexual diseases and gambling are for the most part either romanticized or ignored by the media and kept out of the public eye. Hence, most people are systematically kept unaware of true dangers of vices in our lives (By the way, riding your motorcycle without a helmet makes you very popular with the organ procurement agencies; "Donor Cycle" is the name, and the adage goes, "Give your kid a motorcycle for his 18th birthday, and it's the last gift he'll ever need" - because he will be dead before 19.).

No one can stop a bad habit until he or she really decides a will to stop, thus most court-ordered rehabilitation programs are a waste of taxpayer money. Until the person actually wants to change and end substance abuse, taxpayer money is wasted on the revolving door of laughable "rehab" until a tragedy happens, at which time another brief media blitz strikes (like throwing gasoline on the fire), then all is forgotten, except for the lives destroyed by the media blitz.

Yet, if a person really wants rehabilitation from a destructive vice, it is often very difficult to get help and quite expensive; I guess the difficulty in getting help is that all the resources are tied up pandering to those who belong in jail rather than a rehab unit. Current popular opinion is to condemn the "war on drugs," but the sad fact is you cannot win a war by using taxpayer dollars to fund both sides of the war. We have seen firsthand regarding political talk in one direction and guns being sent to drug lords in the other direction. The other thing is that a war against a vice is different than a war against a physical aggressor grabbing your land and enslaving your people and needs to be fought differently. In short, we have developed a system whereby people with substance addiction problems seeking help cannot get help and those just scamming the rehab route to dodge a jail term get all the benefits. We have also seen a system whereby on one end the U.S. government talks tough about stopping drugs from crossing our borders but actually allows drugs and drug-dealers access to America. The subsequent response is to then militarize the police more, which only leads to animosity between citizens and police, which makes an ideal situation for criminals to operate. After all, when citizens do not trust the political leaders and police, they are not going to confide in the authorities, and crimes will go unreported. Of course, many of the same politicians want to talk tough about human trafficking, but allow illegal aliens easy access. You cannot allow illegal aliens unrestricted access into this country and expect to hinder human trafficking, because it is the undocumented humans that are easiest to traffic, exploit and abuse. Sadly, during the Obama administration, when persons in Utah released a list of illegals, it was the persons releasing the list and not the illegals who were in trouble.

Those are issues where thoughtful analysis could more rationally allocate resources in reasonable proportion to actual risks facing society and good journalistic investigation could impose accountability against the political double speak, which would serve the public well.

Chapter 31
Medical Hype and Public Policy

Since the book "House of God" was written, there has been a myriad of regulations and paperwork hurdles regarding accreditation, authorization, compliance and payment issues, to name a very few. One minor error can get you labeled a Medicare or Medicaid cheater. Everything can get you criminalized and anything can be an excuse not to pay for your patient care services. Thus, the average cost per patient has gone up, regulations have become more cumbersome and salaries have gone down or not kept up with inflation; small wonder almost no one can afford to go into primary care. Also, there is the possibility that any charity work you do can violate a Medicare or Medicaid agreement and make you a criminal. The really smart people have avoided medicine and gone into finance.

The understanding of the interaction of life, death and medicine is also important, because public policy has been influenced by it. For example, the article "To Err is Human" is often cited regarding justification of oppressive enforcement of public policy in healthcare, but the article and references cited did not account for patients with nothing to gain by hospitalizations. When searching for the actual article, I, a seasoned physician, had difficulty obtaining firsthand information and initially could only find access to the summary statements and not the raw article data. If this is the most important research data of my lifetime driving public health policy, why is access so difficult to get to the primary article and data? Further searching did find a copy of "To Err is Human"at http://www,nap.edu/catalog/9728.html. Of interest, the 1999 number of medical errors indicated are not real numbers of medical errors, but extrapolated numbers based mostly on limited studies, such as "Incidence of

Adverse Events and Negligence in Hospitalized Patients —
Results of the Harvard Medical Practice Study I" by Troyen
A. Brennan, M.P.H., M.D., J.D., et al. N Engl J Med 1991;
324:370-376 February 7, 1991, utilizing 1984 New York
hospital data, which itself had extrapolated results. The
figures from table 1 of the Brennan article indicate 30,195
charts located for review, 1278 adverse events occurred
and 306 were due to negligence, a 4% rate of total adverse
events and 1% negligence in 1984 (not 1991, when the
article was published and not 1999 when the Institute of
Medicine study was published) and most of the adverse
events did not cause any long-term sequela. While we
would like the medical error rate to be as close to zero as
humanely possible, I remind people that a manufacturer
with around a 1% to 4% failed product rate is considered
fantastic, and a baseball player getting a hit over 30% of
the time becomes a hall of famer. Hence the standards for
errors are already much tighter in medicine than all other
industries, as it should be. In medicine and surgery
anything over a 0.5% to 1% complication rate is being
evaluated for improvement and those habits were
practiced long before "To Err is Human" was published. I
am certain patient care in 1999, was not the same as in
1984, when the data was originally acquired and am not
comfortable with one NY east coast hospital representing
the entire nation. <u>The Brennan article</u> was interested in
statewide medical errors, thus <u>included **adverse events**
before the index hospitalization</u>, which likely inflated the
hospitalization adverse event rate reported in "Too Err is
Human" because of propagation of extrapolated numbers
to New York state by the Brennan publication and
subsequent extrapolation to the entire U.S
hospitalizations in "Too Err is Human." Hence, even well-
intentioned people need to be careful using older,
retrospective data, evaluating different focus populations,
extrapolating from such diverse data when setting
mandates.

Once we are so ill and near death or in a persistent vegetative state, the risk/ benefit relationship is way off kilter. Even in a low risk situation if there is no (zero) benefit, then the risk/benefit ratio is mathematically "undefined." As the benefit in the denominator of the equation approaches zero, the equation asymptotically approaches infinity for risk. The situation is worse if there is some definable risk, as the risk portion of the equation approaches infinity somewhat faster. Above all, do no harm (aka *primum non nocere* – "first do no harm" or to cite the Hippocratic Oath, "abstain from doing harm"). Certainly, in treating such patients, there is only risk and no benefit, the likelihood for medical error is skewed and should not be part of the data, or should certainly be adjusted for.

Chapter 32
Dirty Little Secrets:
Forced Obligation of all U.S. Doctors to the Organ Procurement Program

Many people do not realize that operating a hospital in the United States requires a lot of "compliance" with regulations, including actively assisting the organ procurement program. Pre-med, medical students, and many doctors were not informed until there was no turning back either. Having legislation or hospital policy forcing the staff to contact Lifebanc regarding every death in the hospital is wrong.

If someone wants to be an organ donor that is their choice; we should also honor their choice not to be an organ donor and not try to pry their organs from them anyhow by going around the dead person and contacting his or her family.

A neurologist told us of a story where a patient had Guillain-Barre and was erroneously pronounced dead, and he began developing tears in his eyes during the organ harvesting process. The procedure was immediately halted. Scary to think a condition that may require the need for temporary respirator support could end you up in the organ donor list instead of the list of survivors.

Brain dead donors are ideal (dead brain, but still beating heart). A difficulty with determining "brain death" is there is no consistent standard. Some places use lack of a perceptible Electroencephalogram (EEG) signal, some use lack of blood flow seen on ultrasound in both carotid arteries, others use lack of blood flow on a nuclear medicine scan. Many medications can suppress EEG signals, and if connections and gain parameters are not adequate, a signal cannot be detected, but the non-detection may not equal death, so one must be very cautious and use many physical and monitoring parameters to make the call with confidence.

The organ procurement program I am familiar with from my training is called Lifebanc. From the Lifebanc website, the mission of Lifebanc is "To increase organ and tissue donation for those awaiting transplant."

Organ procurement has managed to infiltrate society through political back doors. Lifebanc is not only sanctioned by the U.S. government, but hospitals and physicians must participate in Lifebanc/organ procurement to exist. That's right – If a hospital refuses to participate in Lifebanc, it loses all government funding, not just funding for transplant programs, but all funding. The government will not pay for a Medicare patient's knee replacement or a Medicaid patient's prenatal care if the hospital does not contribute to the organ donation business.

A potential organ donor is usually acutely severely ill or injured. The patient's condition is dire, bordering on life and death and probably tending to imminent death. Dead organs cannot be transplanted. Thus, the organs need perfusion, either by a beating heart or by placing the patient on extracorporeal circulation. This means that someone has a beating heart, alive by definition, up until the organs are harvested. When the extraction of usable parts is complete, the patient is killed by medication to stop the heart or switching off the perfusion equipment.

How does an organization, which by legal definition kills people, get the approval of our country's leaders? When organ donation is publicized, the pictures show smiling children whose lives are apparently saved by organ donation. The philosophy is that "The Ends Justify the Means" – but we ultimately live and die within the means. The organ donation propaganda does not show the alcoholic who gets a new liver transplant, nor the brain-injured motorcycle (aka Donor Cycle) rider with his organs ripped from his torso or his de-boned legs flopping off the autopsy table like a piece of boneless chicken.

I speak from experience. During my Student Pathology Fellowship year, I had to perform an autopsy on a person with his eyes and bone marrow harvested. There was a plastic cap in each eye socket. His bones were tore from his lower extremities from the anterior iliac bone to the talus (deboned from hip through the ankle). His legs were sutured with the surgical equivalent of twine. It was ghastly, I wretched and vomited and wretched several times more throughout the autopsy. This was one of 14 autopsies I conducted, and the only one I got sick over. Viewing an organ-harvested body was the determining factor driving me away from pathology. I had performed and assisted on autopsies of neonates, cancer patients and even a mentally ill person who immolated with gasoline, but the organ-harvested body was the most horrifying. Organ procurement propaganda does not mention the occasional accidental near harvesting or maybe even harvesting of organs from very much alive Guillain-Barre, persistent vegetative state, catatonic or "locked in syndrome" patients. Evidently neither do the so called "free press" in the U.S. or politicians ask such questions.

The propagandized myth of organ donation is that every child is saved and lives happily after. The reality is that every transplant patient requires suppression of the immune system to avoid the natural process rejecting a foreign body. This immune suppression results in essentially iatrogenic AIDS. Thus, the transplant patient requires lifelong monitoring and interventions, and the slightest sniffle could represent something life threatening. Unfortunately, the people who know the truth are not talking. The other myth is that the person is dead before donating organs. The fact is, a person is "near death" when they donate organs, the procurement team ultimately ends the life by stopping a beating heart, or ceasing extracorporeal circulation.

The process of organ donation affects healthcare decisions. Often these life and death decisions are made through a resident physician already impaired by severe chronic sleep deprivation deemed too horrible for prisoners of war. It is a chance for someone to be worth more dead than alive. If this one biker dies, we can harvest a bunch of organs that can help several other people, not to mention make a lot of money; I said don't mention the money. Which means when a person goes to the hospital for care, the first decision is whether to treat you or let your condition decline and go to the possible organ donor pool. Since there are many orders of magnitude more possible recipients than donors, your life is worth more dead than alive. Nowadays, when a doctor says, "We don't think he'll make it" you will have to wonder if your family member is really that critically ill or the regional organ procurement program needs to fill a quota.

In the autopsy I previously mentioned, the patient was transferred from an outside rural hospital to a larger metropolis healthcare center. At the major hospital, he was placed in the ER hallway (It was a busy night.), and Lifebanc was contacted. I am not sure if the patient was transferred for the express purpose of organ donation or if his son thought his father was actually going to be cared for at the metropolis facility. My impression from the notes seemed to indicate the physicians at the remote location may have thought the patient would be better served at a more advanced facility, but my review of the chart of the recipient hospital seemed that salvaging the patient's life was not even considered an option and that it was accepted fact the patient was merely there for organ procurement. Talk about a possible horrific miscommunication?

Healthcare resources are tremendously taxed by organ transplantation. If everyone who could use an organ transplant obtains one, the medical system would probably siphon off the entire wealth of our country, perhaps the entire wealth of the world, causing national or international bankruptcy in the quest for immortality. Lifebanc does not tell you that a liver transplant consumes 80 to 300 units of blood products, which is a major contributor to blood shortage for other medical and surgical interventions and causes blood shortages for acute trauma patients and perhaps blood product shortages for cancer patients. Is healthcare economically and socially better to use 80 to 300 units of blood to save dozens to hundreds of lives or a couple lives? You do the math.

Lifebanc does not deal in honesty; it deals in organ procurement. The organization works covertly. For example, while I was a medical student, a representative from Lifebanc indicated in the State of Ohio choosing "Yes" to organ donation on your driver's license means you will be an organ donor if the circumstances of your demise permit. But, if you chose "No" to organ donation on your Ohio driver's license, you are a treated as a "Maybe," which means your family still will be approached for your organs, and despite your wishes you may become an organ donor anyway. The representative from Lifebanc did not indicate if the family would be informed of your "No" to organ donation designation on your license or not. Obviously, no one voted for that interpretation of "Yes" and "No." Not only does interpreting "no" as "maybe" manipulate the organ procurement system, but reinterpreting "no" in a political and legal context probably goes a long way to allowing many criminals, sexual molesters and rapists go free, plea bargain to lesser charges, or go on to have a prestigious political career.

One transplant physician stated to our medical school class that "people should not be allowed to have a driver's license or healthcare in this country if they do not agree to participate in organ donation," I was flabbergasted. Had I known this, I never would have chosen a career in medicine. That militant attitude regarding one's societal obligation to organ procurement did turn me away from my undergraduate aim of being a transplant surgeon.

Here is an example of some of the legislative code regarding organ procurement compliance. "42 CFR 482.45 – Condition of participation: Organ, tissue, and eye procurement of the 1996 Health Insurance Portability and accountability act requires any facility participating in seeing patients insured under any government healthcare plan to have and implement written protocols that Incorporate an agreement with an organ procurement organization (OPO), under which it must notify, in a timely manner, the OPO or a third party designated by the OPO of individuals whose death is imminent or who have died in the hospital, incorporate an agreement with at least one tissue bank and at least one eye bank, ensure, in collaboration with the designated OPO, that the family of each potential donor is informed of its options to donate or to decline to donate, ensure that the hospital works cooperatively with the designated OPO, tissue bank and eye bank in educating staff on donation issues, reviewing death records to improve identification of potential donors, and maintaining potential donors while necessary testing and placement of potential donated organs, tissues, and eyes take place. The individual designated by the hospital to initiate the request to the family must be an organ procurement representative or a designated requestor".

Under "HIPAA 164.512 Uses and disclosures for which an authorization or opportunity to agree or object is not required," no written authorization is required by patient or family regarding organ procurement notification. This is not a horror movie plot, or is it? This is federal law, an act of Congress, and evidenced by the 2004 "Organ Donation and Recovery Improvement Act." It's not going away anytime soon. Further information can be obtained by reading an article on the Hospice Patients Alliance website, by Paul Byrne, MD titled "Do Your Organs Belong To The Government." Physicians' hands are tied. If they do not participate in organ procurement referrals, they risk not being able to practice medicine in this country, or many other countries, which is a huge cost after you are locked in by 7-12 years of medical training beyond college and several hundreds of thousands of dollars in student loan debt, or have your VISA status or citizenship processing dependent on your compliance. The problem is even greater as less private healthcare is available and the government plays a bigger role in our lives. Unless there is an immediate major change, nothing is yours, not even your organs.

Why does the clergy allow this horrifying situation to happen and remain speechless? The Catholic Church claims to value life by denouncing abortion, yet accepts organ harvesting. Does the Catholic Church and other religions selectively apply the End Justifies the Means philosophy? An organized religion considers killing a fetus unacceptable for stem cell research to possibly help a life, but tolerates, even embraces killing an injured adult to harvest organs in attempt to possibly help a life? This sounds like a rather inconsistent valuation of life to me. I suspect the religious agencies also have been duped by the organ procurement industry propaganda, which focuses on the organ recipient, convinces everyone the donor is "essentially dead," and ignores the procurement process that requires stopping a beating heart. No legitimate religion could endorse the selective systematic killing of one patient to save another; such a situation essentially declares "all lives are not equal" and that religions do not respect life. What part of "Thou Shall Not Kill" aren't people getting?

Finally, the organ procurement system is corrupt. In attempt to avoid corruption, there are objective transplant list criteria, but as has been seen the list is malleable under influence of political power and money. For example, in North Carolina, the allocation of organs did not always follow the plan. In a well publicized case many years ago an American was left to die because of being bumped from the transplant list. The daughter of an exploited illegal immigrant was given higher priority than an American citizen, because a wealthy builder contacted a certain politician (called in a favor) who managed to apply her influence to subvert the transplant list. What is worse is that the girl died, an American died, the physician was tied up in malpractice litigation, and the politician and businessman were never held accountable for their role in undermining the organ donation transplant system. It can and will happen again. As long as such perverse greed and self-indulgence are unaccountable in this country there will be no limit to the ability of the rich, powerful and politically connected to manipulate the organ procurement and transplant process to their advantage at a whim. Why can everyone manipulate the healthcare system without accountability, except the physicians actually trained in healthcare?

Within the background of misrepresentation and behind the scenes manipulation do realize that your organ donation may be an ultimate act of love and forgiveness, because for the most part your organs are not likely to go to some innocent child, or one with a rare congenital disease, but statistically more likely to go to those who already had their chance and screwed up their organs by bad habits. Your organs may go to the drug lord who killed your other family members; it may go to someone whose values are radically different from your own. Your organ may go to a deserving person awaiting transplant on the list or may go to someone with money and influence to get a politician to help cut into the line. You have to be willing to forgive all such situations in being a fully consenting donor. Only organ donation and abortion are granted immunity from "Informed Consent" practices and seem to systematically avoid truly informed consent. Get a hangnail surgery, and all the discussions including the incredibly rare possibility of death is mentioned, but Democrat politicians seem to want women to think abortion is akin to choosing between Chiclets versus gummy bears and organ procurement moves stealthily in the political background undermining your rights to your own physical organs.

The organ harvesting industry should be halted until there is true informed consent – (like showing the mutilated body of an organ donor), there must be honest assessment of the true costs of organ donation in consuming resources from other treatments. People should be informed the majority of organ recipients are not just the cute children exploited in the commercials. Manipulation of the transplant system from politicians must end, and there must be serious accountability for trying to manipulate the transplant list. Finally, Lifebanc and other organ procurement systems need to cease covert activities that infiltrate the government funding process and stop interpreting a "no" as "maybe". Only then can persons appropriately decide under truly "informed consent" if they want their organs harvested.

Chapter 33
No Such Thing as Good
Samaritan Legal Protection

You may have heard of "Good Samaritan Laws." The more accurate description of the law is a good deed may still be punished. You hear it often enough – someone does something really great but broke a company policy so is fired. You name it, a clever lawyer can find an angle to sue over it. While working in HVAC I heard a news story on the radio of a criminal trying to steal a furnace from a construction site only to sue the builder and heating company for his back injury during the theft, and there was a story regarding a burglar suing the homeowner because the criminal tripped on something and injured himself.

Same thing happens in medicine, so just because a law seems to imply legal protection for being a great human and doing something good and wonderful, don't believe it. This is a shame, because these breaches of the sanctity of the Good Samaritan Laws discourage people from helping others in times of need and make for a worse nation. As I indicated earlier, if you make a weapon to slaughter a whole community, you are internationally exempted from prosecution, but injure a person trying to remove them from a burning vehicle and your life is destroyed.

I mention this because it happens and everyone needs to be aware. Good Samaritan Laws are fickle, sometimes protecting any rescue person and other times only protecting trained rescue workers, who are in a volunteer capacity and other times, protecting no one. My take is to help if you can despite the obvious legal risks. The point is Good Samaritan Laws are state laws, not federal laws, and subject to political and legal whimsy. Do not feel a false sense of security because of an apparent Good Samaritan Law. Sadly now, you can understand why some people chose not to help. Rescue workers have been sued for allegedly causing spine injuries, and the fallout is that even the most minor injury often results in many people unnecessarily getting strapped to a backboard and going to the ED; some of the procedure is extra caution, some is medical-legal waste of resources. The lack of evidence proving efficacy of using a backboard in suspected spine injury, even citing a study indicating worse outcome using a backboard, is described in "The Evidence against Backboards" article by Bryan E. Bledsoe, DO, FACEP, FAAEM on AUG 1, 2013. The fallout of adapting hospital policy to lawsuits came to embarrassing extremes, told to me by my mother, a former hospital secretary. A patient fell in a hospital parking lot a few feet from the entrance. The emergency room was nearby. Hospital policy at that time utilizing medical legal precautionary advice led to an ambulance call. Thus, the patient, only a few feet from a hospital entrance, waited for an ambulance to come, assess, place on a stretcher, and transfer him to the adjacent emergency room. The situation would have been an even more sadly comedic if the ambulance took the person to a different hospital. Of course, the media came, and in typical "throw gasoline on a fire" form created a blame circus. Apparently, all the negative publicity led the hospital administrators to do some serious screaming and blaming of state regulators and legal system that set up such a situation to begin with. Damned if you do and damned if you don't – pick your poison, do you want to be slandered, libeled and sued for trying to help or for not trying to help, but you will be slandered, libeled and sued. Just another example of people trying to do good getting punished, but people who make weapons of mass destruction are exempted.

Chapter 34
My Perspective of Healthcare Bureaucracy

During the 2008 Democrat Primary debates, a question was asked regarding the Iraq War Memo, justifying the cause of invading Iraq in 2003. The question was "Did you read the Iraq War Memo?" The answer of most the Democrat politicians, including lead candidates Hillary Clinton and John Edwards, was "I was briefed," which means the answer was, "No, I did not read the memo." So here was perhaps the most important memo of the decade, if not the last quarter century, and most likely the most important memo of their political careers, millions of lives would be impacted, yet these Democrat candidates for the presidency of the United States of America did not read the memo. I guess going to war, killing hundreds of thousands of enemy soldiers, killing tens of thousands of civilians, and displacing millions of persons, was not worth reading. Only Mr. Obama and Mr. Kucinich claimed to have actually read the war memo, and they were of the minority who voted "No" to invading Iraq. Maybe more politicians should have read the memo.

While I understand a politician cannot read and mull over the consequences of every word in every political document, I do expect the major ones to at least be briefly viewed. If something as important as going to war or not, is not important enough for a politician, especially a Democrat politician to read, then I suspect they do not read much of anything presented before them. It is shameful that illiteracy and the ability to claim complete ignorance appears to be a virtue, which enhances a Democrat's political career.

So, while I, like many, considered a need for healthcare reform, it was rather disappointing to think such an important legislation plan for restructuring healthcare in America would never be read, or even briefly glanced at, by the very people voting the plan into policy. The so-called Affordable Care Act (another cute political name meaning exactly the opposite of its name) was completely constructed as a mechanism to divert taxpayer funds for political favors and is not affordable, nor has much to do with improving healthcare – it was complete pork barrel politics at its worst. Also, anytime someone who actually did read the documents raised objections to the incongruities and unintended consequences (or perhaps intended consequences), those objections were immediately crushed by the political propaganda machine that we in the United States call the "news." The United States' so-called "free press" (another misleading political name that really means, "propaganda machine") has a lot of nerve stating Pravda is propaganda.

Hence, all sensible objections to the healthcare plan or portions of the seriously flawed plan were absolutely crushed and dismissed.

As a person who has lived life, from both inside and outside the medical realm, I knew what I liked and disliked about healthcare in the United States and contacted several politicians regarding healthcare policy. Of course, being an American citizen, none of my ideas were ever seriously considered. Typically, Republican politicians never even responded to my letters, and Democrat politicians sent a form letter thanking me for my "interest in this serious issue" facing millions of people, but never really gave any indication they actually read the letter. I guess the stereotypes that Democrats don't read and Republicans don't care is true.

In the process of trying to contact politicians about healthcare policy, even before the 2008 elections, and in later sending my proposals to President Obama's healthcare advisor before the ACA was completed, I learned how little an American citizen can do for America. We are thwarted at every attempt to have meaningful contact with a politician.

First, as an American citizen, you are only allowed to contact your immediate congressional and senate representatives. Even then your contact information for constituency is not enough. You have to follow their fixed format or be rejected. For example, your name address and zip code are not enough, you must have ZIP+4 zip code or you cannot contact your politician via the official website; a minor inconvenience to be sure, but a barrier to communication between elected official and constituent nonetheless.

Second, no matter how important an issue is to you, or how much of an expert you think you are or actually are, if your representative is not on the committee dealing with the subject, you have no input into American politics. Everything in American politics is done by committee; if your representative is not on the committee, you have no representation on that committee. Many issues live or die in committee. No American citizen is allowed to contact the committee directly and American citizens do not get to vote who is on a given committee. There is not necessarily particular expertise of the politician related to the focus of a given committee, so essentially committee members can be relatively ignorant of the topics of their committee and only obtain invited advice. Not uncommonly, such advice is provided by persons with a vested interest in the outcome. In other words, your vote matters little because all agendas to be voted upon are first raised or buried in committee before your elected representatives actually gets to consider and vote on the issue. Hence democracy has been usurped by committee system.

Now I note that when Soviet Georgia tried to forcibly annex Ossetia in 2008, those foreign representatives did have an audience with both Sens. John McCain and Joe Biden. Hence, foreigners have access to U.S. political leaders, which is denied to American citizens. Of course, that "access" did include about $250,000 to each senator to purchase influence, and it worked, because both Mr. Biden and Mr. McCain publically pronounced how horrible Russia was in stopping Soviet Georgia's forced annexation of Ossetia. Money talks.

The issue of money talking makes an even greater impact when you realize that as of 2010 statistics the United States has a debt to GDP (debt/productivity) ratio over 100%, which means we take on more debt than we can afford. When you realize only Greece, which went through bankruptcy, and Japan have a higher debt to productivity ratio, it is scary. Yes, all those "at risk" European Union nations like Italy, Ireland, Spain etc. all had more productivity with respect to their debt than the United States, they just have smaller economies and are also somewhat constrained by not having an individual currency to adjust accordingly, as they are in a common currency market. Japan has about a 200% debt to productivity ratio, which is certainly high, but at least the debt is about 95% or greater owned by Japanese businesses and Japanese citizens. The United States had a full one-third of its debt (33.33%) owned by foreign companies and foreign individuals, which means foreign money can have a significant impact on U.S. elections and U.S. policies.

Against this backdrop, I will indicate what I sent the politicians and why I thought the proposals had at least some merit for consideration. As an aside, for clarification, I will note here that many authors refer to the current managed care model, pre-Affordable Care Act, as a "fee for service" model, which is technically a confusing misnomer, with different meaning than the pre-Managed Care Fee-for-Service model. The current misnomer of fee for service implies you get paid for your services, which is not exactly true. You may get some payment for your services, called reimbursement with prearranged payment schedule for a given service or diagnosis, but that is not the model of sending a reasonable fee for your services and actually getting paid for it. For clarification, in my letter sample below, I mean Fee-for-Service under the pre-managed care model.

This is a representative sample of communication written to one of many politicians, some of the wording was amended in each letter to make it more palatable to politicians of a given political leaning or to address a specific comment a specific politician or party representative may have made, but the proposals and reasons were similar for all politicians attempted to be contacted:

James M Gannon MD:
Proposal for a healthcare bill.
Representative (---),
While my proposal is not a broad scope as your plan, it may be more readily acceptable in the short term. Also it may give you some political momentum as election season approaches.

My observations are based on years of experience as a HVAC service technician covered under various health plans, my experience with student health plans from undergraduate and medical school experience, undergraduate minor in Economics and now from my experiences as a physician.

Under the current Managed Care Healthcare model we spend a greater percentage of a larger GNP than we did *under the old Fee-for-Service model*: You remember that model; patients were cared for and physicians were paid.*

Now the healthcare budget is spent in making barriers to healthcare. If denied long enough, the patients' medical care will fall on a competitor or the government. There is a quandary as hospitals, physicians and insurance companies must compete in a competitive capitalist market for survival, yet make altruistic decisions whenever possible. Companies make more money by denying healthcare than providing it, and doctors make more money on their documentation or business arrangements rather than caring for patients.

Here are the proposals I would like as a Medical Reform Bill:
1. Make insurance a long-term commitment. Form insurer/patient relationships that last several decades. Such an arrangement gives an insurer a vested interest in keeping customers/patients healthy. A specific example why to adopt such a policy is the fact that many student insurance plans, deny routine gynecologic coverage to young women, leaving them to potentially develop cervical cancer on a future employer/insurance carrier's budget.

Corollary supporting my proposal: When the logging industry was granted short-term contracts to a forest, essentially the countryside was raped. With long-term commitments re-forestation has occurred, there is an investment in the future.

2. Standardize healthcare. The "Executive Physical" not only implies but expresses the idea that some lives are more important than others. Give everyone the "Executive Physical," or a reasonable standard of a physical exam for everyone, even executives.

I am aghast that drug addicts on Medicaid have better health benefits than college students, professional students and American workers. This situation has resulted from trying to shut people out of the insurance system, by linking insurance to employment. Unfortunately, as employers trim their budgets by slashing healthcare benefits, the American worker is the one left without insurance.

Essentially there needs to be a philosophical change to accept that all lives are worth saving and a practical understanding that when you try to provide exclusive coverage, well deserving people are shut out.

3. Standardize paperwork. As a very conservative estimate, billions of healthcare dollars, unknown number of trees and millions of potentially productive man-hours are spent by the government and the insurance industry trying to avoid paying legitimate physician fees.

At the present time, a physician must spend 20-40 minutes of paperwork to document a 5-10 minute patient encounter, and if the correct buzzwords are not made the physician is not paid and may even be accused of fraud. It currently takes 1-3 office staff to process insurance paperwork for the first physician; economies of scale take over as more physicians are in the group. Such a paperwork burdensome situation has killed many private medical practices in this country. In the current medical practice setting, much to the chagrin of several disappointed physicians, the patient is the least important factor in healthcare. Physicians are being forced to be businessmen and secretaries ahead of their calling to heal patients.

4. Set up a Usual, Customary and Reasonable fee schedule.
Why should Medicaid pay $350 for a medical service, Medicare pays $500, a private insurer pays $1000 and an individual is billed and expected to pay $5000 for the same service? In other words the price of healthcare

is artificially elevated for individuals, thus making it artifactually unaffordable.

Many of the uninsured people could afford Usual, Customary and Reasonable healthcare costs. Why does an individual worker pay 5-10 times what the multimillion-dollar insurance companies or the multibillion-dollar government pays? We are pricing healthcare, not nuts and bolts. The price of health services should not be determined as if one were giving a quantity discount in the hardware industry.

5. Forget the old days where insurance was given as a condition of employment. When I was a high school student working in the grocery store, I had my own personal health insurance through work, even though I was only 16-17 years old and still covered under my parent's healthcare policies. Companies which do provide health insurance typically find the cheapest policy, which leaves tens of millions of workers underinsured.

During my medical Internship year, I met a patient working three part-time jobs without health insurance, while a cocaine addict in the room across the hall had full Medicaid coverage.

In summary long-term investment in the patient, standardization of paperwork and services, fair prices and opportunities for everyone to be insured will solve this crisis.

The government, insurance industry, hospitals, physicians and patients all have a vested interest in our healthcare system and need to work together.

My plan would provide the practical foundation for making healthcare more efficient, affordable and easier to participate in for all parties.

Sincerely,

James M Gannon MD.

Those were my thoughts. Point 4 of my letter actually indicates that at least a portion of the "healthcare crisis" was man-made (i.e. politician-made) by unjust billing and collection policies and the laws that force such policies.

My point was to emphasize that the healthcare quagmire had become so bad, that the last job of a doctor anymore was taking care of patients. Perhaps that is why I love medical mission work so much – we just focus on patient care as best we can. Nowadays, the first three duties a physician needs to be concerned with is "compliance," "compliance" and compliance. You must comply with Federal laws, various state laws which occasionally may even overtly conflict with federal law and comply with hospital policies that are much more Draconian, as "hospital policies" are designed to ensure that the merest appearance of non-compliance is avoided. You must have preemptive documentation to prove your innocence – or you are guilty.

After compliance, compliance and compliance, you must then focus on billing. If a doctor does not document absolutely correctly, the bill is not paid. Yes, every insurance company and government unit is pre-absolved of all responsibility for errors and lies and the physician and hospital are ultimately responsible for everything. Being held responsible for the action of other people over whom you have no control is inherently wrong too, but that is a medical practice fact. Yes, almost every government paper and insurance document contain the phrase "authorization for the visit or procedure does not guarantee payment for services rendered." So not only must you document billing correctly or you will not be paid, but even documenting correctly and performing the appropriate service above the best standards does not guarantee payment. The other aspect of billing is that if you bill the wrong code, you are a criminal. If you bill the correct code, the government and private insurance companies will look for ways to "down code" (pay less), but if you bill too little you are a fraud looking for favors, and if you bill too much you are a thief. Billing is very important.

Billing schematics are no small part of why healthcare is so expensive. For example, based on a true scenario, a psychologist would see private pay out of pocket patients for $40 each visit. Patient comes in once a month. You see, healthcare is not free and not cheap but is affordable. Eventually the group practice decided to take Medicaid patients. That particular state's Medicaid program contains a fairly common language stating they must get the most favorable rate of billing (aka get billed the least). This is not "pay the least," it is "Billed the least." Also, Medicaid programs have an "all in clause," so either everyone or no one in a given group sees Medicaid patients. And you thought you lived in a free country. Some programs of government and insurance will pay based on a fixed rate for the visit, regardless what is actually billed. Hence, one may bill $120 for an office visit or $3000 a day for a hospital stay, but the government or insurer pays $35 for the doctor's office visit and $250 a day for a hospital stay. The problem is that the uninsured individual is legally obligated to pay $120 for the doctor office visit that all the insurers get for much less and pay the full $3000 a day for a hospital bed. Hence the insurance game drives up the cost for the uninsured and an uncomfortable but affordable actual cost of healthcare becomes a ludicrous hospital bill that could bankrupt many people.

Sometimes the private insurance or government programs pay a percentage of what is billed. If a program like Medicaid pays 10% of what it is billed, no one can afford to operate a business under such circumstances, so the facility must either bill higher or not see Medicaid patients. For example, if a doctor wants $100, he or she must bill Medicaid $1000 (10% of $1,000 is $100). Again, the result is the private person is now expected to pay $1000 for the $100 service. In my above example, Medicaid was paying about $30-40 for a psychology visit, but it took a bill of about $120 to get that $30 dollars or so. Because of legal constraints, when the group decided to take Medicaid patients, under the contract "lowest bill conditions," it means that the psychologist could no longer legally offer $40 consultation sessions to private individuals, for Medicaid was being billed $120, even though Medicaid may have actually paid the same $40 or less. The Medicaid contract, if taken to rigid extremes, could also indicate that if you do charity work, or give a patient an unbilled visit for any reason, then you are a criminal violating the Medicaid contract.

In prior days physician offices were very forgiving of a patient not being able to afford the co-pay: "You cannot spare the $20? Don't worry about it." Now that situation of debt forgivenes can be considered Medicare and Medicaid fraud. Private insurers want a reimbursement, too. The logic under a given example is that if the payment for a physician service was $100 and insurance paid $80 and the patient paid $20, all was OK. Yet if the doctor stated to the patient, "Don't worry about the co-pay," then the insurance company would want a re-calculation stating then the services were not worth $100, but were only worth $80. Hence insurance will readjust and pay you $64, and the patient expected to pay the other $16. So, you can see that a compassionate physician can get really screwed over by the insurance companies or can be accused of fraud by the government. The end result is that doctors are essentially legally coerced into sending unpaid co-pays to collections to comply with legal and civil contractual obligations. Such a situation drives a wedge between doctor-patient relationships, which is perhaps the political aim. To iterate the greatest political-media coup: Convincing people doctors are the bad guys and the politicians are the good guys.

Now you see that compliance, compliance, compliance, billing (including billing compliance) and documentation all take precedence over patient care.

If you did not document it, it never happened. No, physical reality does not count in the medical-legal world, unless it can be used against you. The obvious fact that you physically did something means nothing. For example, if a surgeon performs an appendectomy, the fact of the surgery operating room time, patient scar and pathology specimen documenting an appendix means nothing without an operative note. Now, if the patient had a bad complication and sued, the lack of an operative note will not protect the surgeon. In short, anything you say or do not say can be used against you, but only what has been prospectively documented can be used in your favor.

As indicted above, many things take precedence over patient care in the healthcare system. The Health Information Portability and Accountability Act (HIPAA) also has had, detrimental impact on patient care and has been a devastating piece of legislation destroying the doctor-patient relationship. HIPAA has restricted effective communication regarding patient care. It is such a punitive piece of legislation that almost two decades since inception we were only beginning the "portability" aspect of the law. There are attempts at regional medical record keeping, but you lose access if you do not use the system frequently and the utilization still requires a special additional patient authorization of medical release statement for the regional database information to be legally accessed, even if you do have technical access and a solid patient care reason to view the information. Hence, the portability aspect of HIPAA is still not very portable. If a patient has a psychiatric history, another special warning box in the computer demands you declare why you want access to the chart and has you provide your login and password. Seriously, I wanted to look at the chest complaint illness medical history to correlate with a chest X-ray and stumbled across a chart with a psychiatric history and the warning box – do you say forget it or do you risk accessing the chart and getting fired? In other words, there are sources of resistance to having doctors access medical charts for the patients they are supposed to be caring for, I consider that situation seriously flawed. Unfortunately, even more punitive aspects of HIPAA have evolved such that even a near breach of information is treated as if the breach actually happened. So, the more recent focus on "portability" – even with all its problems – will again take a back seat to "accountability." In 2014 I received a piece of mail documenting and "certifying" my dental insurance status for the past five years. I had assumed the document was related to the more recent so-called Affordable Care Act, but it actually stated it was required by 1996 HIPAA law. So, HIPAA clauses were kicking in in 2014?

Everyone in healthcare is on a "need to know basis," which means nurses second guessing prescriptions written or not written, because the nurses do not have access to documentation regarding issues the doctor already adressed. Families have been denied access to the patient, because any accidental allowing of the wrong person to know something is a crime. The societal fabric of neighbors caring for neighbors has been ripped to shreds. People must now convalesce and die in abject loneliness, because merely answering a question like "How's John been?" can lead to immediate dismissal from your job, criminal charges and usury fines. I was a lowly medical student when a unit clerk was looking puzzled holding the phone trying to decide if anyone should talk to the person on the other end or not, because she was worried about HIPAA. The seriousness of the unit clerk's predicament is only fully appreciated when considering a tragic event many years later in the suicide of a London hospital nurse very shortly after violating hospital privacy policy regarding a prank call inquiring on the condition of the Duchess of Cambridge. Remember, it is not only the legal consequences directly from the government, but the company continually reinforced threats to workers in response to a given law that rules an employee's world. Even if a law is eventually ruled unconstitutional, violating a company policy is indefensible. One of our secretaries was queried by administration for accessing and printing patient reports for our department chair. If obtaining information through the myriad of databases was too complex, he would ask the skilled secretary to retrieve relevant reports. It was all legitimate access for providing optimal patient care, but the secretary was threatened with possible termination until the chairman cleared up the issue. Much like a Stalin-era Soviet communist community, no one is talking and everything you do is monitored.

Things like Joint Commission on Accreditation of Healthcare Organizations (JCAHO or aka "joint commission") cost healthcare a huge amount and accomplish very little. For example, a patient needed a fairly urgent central line placed while I was in medical school. We put in an order for the line, and four hours later, no line. I walked down to central services, and they had no idea if the order was ever processed or not, so I requested they just "give me a line for the patient now and I'll take it up with me." Four hours to get a STAT order processed is horrific but nowhere does JCAHO measure such processes. Thus, JCAHO jumps on the flavor of the year for what simple to measure elements are available (like if the exact time and date in the exact format have been clearly written in the chart or if the ordering doctors name is both hand-written and printed in the chart). The redundancy of both printing and writing your name in the chart, just takes more time away from patient care. This has nothing to do with patient care, but is chart supervision of whatever political medical whim has blown at that time period. In other words, much organization oversight measures simple to measure items, not issues of importance. Hence, for the most part, issues or processes JCAHO can measure are quite limited and occasionally useless to patient care. Perhaps some JCAHO metrics are useful, they can speak for themselves, but from a physician point of view JCAHO is just another layer of expensive bureaucracy due to the managed care environment. In a free market system, bad doctors or facilities will be forced to improve or lose patients to others. In managed care, the patient is a fixed commodity, so only bureaucratic regulation can be used, which is the least efficient allocation of improvement methods. The only thing I ever noticed from JCAHO visits were a lot of nervous short-tempered administrators who cared more about where you placed your coffee cup than if you delivered appropriate patient care, and new paint on the walls. Of course, no one ever asks if any of the myriad of regulatory agencies at various public and private levels actually improves patient care, because that would require goals, accountability and consequences, which may infringe on the inherent bureaucratic belief that more regulation is always better.

While I know there needs to be some standards and should be reasonable protection of personal information, I do not think we need to hamstring medical communication and bankrupt the system under excessive regulation. After all, doctors and nurses are human but are also professionally trained human beings dedicated to caring for people. Hence, our dedication to helping others already leads to inherent interest in making healthcare better for each and every patient. Dehumanizing the workforce and taking the focus away from patient care, no matter how well-intentioned, cannot be good for the patient.

In summary, the evolution of healthcare in my lifetime went from a system where every worker was insured, to only full-time white-collar workers or fortunate union blue collar workers had healthcare benefits, to a time where too many working Americans are uninsured, but the healthcare expenses of drug addicts and persons in this country illegally are covered by the taxpayer. Under the same time period, we went from a program where physicians and facilities were actually paid for the services they rendered and patients could choose any doctor and any place they like for medical care, to a system where patients had no choice in healthcare providers and most the money in healthcare was spent making barriers to paying for medical services provided. During this transition, patient care declined, cost of care (at least billings) went up astronomically and regulation increased dramatically.

Chapter 35
The Failures of the Affordable Care Act

Within the aforementioned background information: Enter political discussions and the Affordable Care Act.

The Affordable Care Act is a long document of thousands of pages, whereby the only persons who actually read the legislation were those opposed to it and may take generations to work out all the nuances.

The reason most workers lost healthcare benefits was due to a law called The McDonald's Law, during the Reagan era. This law was designed so companies like The McDonald's Corporation and others who hired a lot of part-time minor aged workers did not have to pay for healthcare benefits, especially since those minor aged persons usually already had health insurance under their parents' policies. Well, the fallout was that all part-time workers were excluded from any requirements for employers to supply health insurance or any other benefits. Hence, for the retail industry, the impact of the law led to a reshuffling so most the retail workforce would become "part-time" and healthcare benefits would be removed. The manufacturing adaptation was to provide the benefits, but hire fewer workers and have them work more hours. Obviously, the simple fix would be to repeal or amend such legislation to correct any flaws. After all, Democrats readily blame the Republicans for harming the American worker, yet neither under Mr. Clinton nor Mr. Obama's presidencies while also having majorities in Congress and Senate, did Democrats ever reverse one of those "oppressive Republican schemes."

The only facts we really know about the Affordable Care Act is that it is really expensive (not so affordable) and that a lot of political wheeling and dealing was done by Democrat politicians to get other Democrat politicians to buy into it – or rather getting other Democrat politicians sold into it. We know tens of millions of dollars to billions of dollars for influence changed political hands; in this case, it was an entirely Democrat political exchange of money and influence, because the Republicans essentially sat it out. Supposedly there were healthcare plan proposals from Republican politicians, which were insulted or ignored, much like politicians ignore letters from their constituency on the subject.

In the 2008 Democrat primaries, there was a question regarding healthcare. It was the time where candidate Obama mocked candidate Hillary Clinton's "mandate for all-in the program," yet President Obama pushed for the very "mandate" candidate Obama previously mocked. Dennis Kucinich had the most straightforward answer, which made it the totally unacceptable answer: "Medicare for everyone." While I admittedly prefer market-centered approach indicated by the sample letter I sent to many politicians I can respect Mr. Kucinich's model to achieve the same outcome. I am admittedly suspect of a "one-party payer" system where that payer is an unaccountable government bureaucracy. Seems like a set-up for a Third World political health model. Some politicians try to liken the Affordable Care Act to successful First World socialized medicine in other countries, while simultaneously openly denying the obvious socialism/communism inherent in the plan. Those nations' healthcare plans were not thousands of pages long. In other words, a socialized medicine model may work in a socialist nation, where everything else is socialized, but having a socialized healthcare system while the rest of the country is capitalist has inherent inefficiencies and costs. Healthcare workers pay a capitalist tuition for medical training and capitalist room and board, utilities, transportation and groceries during education years. Doctors training in socialist nations do not have hundreds of thousands of dollars in student loan debt accruing interest while in training. Hospitals have utility bills and labor expenses. The idea that doctors, nurses and hospitals should have capitalist expenses, but socialist reimbursement, is unfair. Thus, making a hybrid system whereby the components and goals are diametrically opposed is not a good idea. Ironically, we saw the obverse of the healthcare situation in how the U.S. banking and auto industry are capitalist with regards to making money, but socialist/communist requiring taxpayer bailouts when they lose money. Although many developed countries have socialized medicine, they generally have much greater waiting times to see a physician or to obtain a given surgery than Americans are accustomed. Finally, some of those socialist nations have been struggling on the verge of bankruptcy and austerity measures, which makes them a questionable model to follow.

Unfortunately, neither my plan nor Mr. Kucinich's idea had the requisite amount of graft, political posturing, favors and kickback to be politically feasible, even if making reasonable economic sense. Neither Mr. Kucinich's views nor my views required several thousands of pages in which to hide information and bury future systemic time bombs.

A good healthcare plan would not punish people for being productive members of society and reward people for being leeches. A good healthcare plan would not punish companies who do society a great good by providing healthcare for their workers and would not punish workers for receiving a benefit they will rarely use most of their lives by enacting extra systematic taxation. I am not sure the Affordable Care Act was a success by any of those measures.

The Affordable Care Act did not repair the fragmented healthcare delivery structure. For example, when I was a child, every working family seemed to have had healthcare. Thus, when a kid fell from a tree and broke his forearm, the child went to the emergency room and got the forearm repaired. Now, there will be a battle where the injured child parent's health insurance refuses to pay. It will require the homeowner's insurance to pay, but the homeowner's insurance will not pay without a fight and will then raise insurance rates on the homeowner. In the interim, there are unpaid bills, threats of legal collections for those bills, and former friends now suing each other, and the victim (kid with the broken arm) being called into question for bad judgment and who is really to blame. What a mess. The same situation happens for car accidents and injuries. In prior days, if you were hurt you got help, but now you get an inquisition: "Was this at home or work?"; "Is it work-related?"; "Will you be filing disability forms?"; "Do you have insurance?"; "Will your homeowners, auto or medical insurance be covering it?" You are supposed to know the answers to all such possible questions in your time of need prior to being treated.

Another aspect of a great – or even good – healthcare plan would be to put the care of the patient first instead of the battle of "Who's going to pay for this?" first. Again, a dismal failure on the part of the Affordable Care Act.

For example, Social Security was supposed to be a retirement plan, not a disability plan or medical plan for politically-selected diseases. Workers Compensation has the nice ideal that if you are injured at work and have no other medical insurance your work-related injuries will be covered. Various government disability plans also have a component of medical treatment in addition to monies received for not being able to work. All the aforementioned examples were potential huge pools of saving money, not tapped by the Affordable Care Act. After all, if everyone is insured, then there is no need for Workers Compensation, the medical aspect of a Disability Claim, and certain disease conditions could be removed from the Social Security budget. These are all tremendous potential cost savings, none of which were realized by the Affordable Care Act.

Finally, Medicaid needs to be addressed. Medicaid was supposed to be a healthcare program for poor people but has turned into a political mess. Honest, hard-working people in a low-paying job without healthcare benefits are too often better off not working so they can get healthcare. Single mothers and the guys that get them pregnant are economically discouraged from working (get a job and lose your child's healthcare; get married, and the child and girl lose health and welfare benefits), so taxpayers must now support such "families." My wife once talked to a young single mother about plans like "What are you going to do with your life?" to which the young mom stated, "Me and my baby got welfare." Is this the new "American Dream," landing a welfare situation? The "welfare" budget is so bloated that people earning more than $40,000 a year in New York State may apply for home heating credits and assistance under "welfare." Medicaid is comprised of many people who are discouraged from being productive members of society, those for whom the American Dream is now, welfare. Medicaid budgets have taxpayers shoulder the expensive medical consequences of substance abusers, while hard working persons get nothing. There are very few "just poor" people getting Medicaid; too many people seem to have some sort of scam and a really bad entitled attitude. A lot of young people going to college are technically "poor" and living on student loans, but do not qualify for Medicaid. Hence, Medicaid is for the "politically poor" classified persons, not actual poor people.

The point is that if everyone is covered on Medicare, then there is no "Us vs. Them" attitude, like Medicaid inherently invokes, and no need for all the duplication of resources by 50 state Medicaid programs that to some degree copy federal Medicare programs anyhow. Then we are truly all one and the same. Medicaid infrastructure could be retained to some extent for the administrative aspects of care locally, but significant savings would have been realized. Instead, the Affordable Care Act robbed the Medicare fund for older retired workers to fill the state Medicaid funds, which re-emphasizes the "Us vs. Them" attitude and leaves American citizens divided and conquered.

Finally, the "all in" mandate clause is a prime example of political hypocrisy at its worst. "All in," except the unions. "All in," except the politicians. The politicians have exempted themselves from Social Security as well, not bad for another example of an "all in" policy. Ironically, the same politicians do not demand their pension system or Government Motors pensions be funded 70 years into the future, as they imposed on the U.S. Postal Service. If the policy is really any good, there should be no exemptions. Again, the Affordable Care Act fails to be a fair, reasonable and uniform application of public policy.

What the Affordable Care Act does accomplish is creating a legal minefield, as it now makes people responsible for actions over which they have no control. For example, if your patients are not happy and satisfied, you can be docked reimbursement for your services. In an era where a lot of people, including polysubstance drug abusers seek opioids and benzodiazepine medications, saying "No" to a drug addict can result in poor patient satisfaction survey results. Hence, being a very good doctor and not pandering into the drug problem cuts a doctor's pay. The Affordable Care Act has increased drug addiction problems in the United States because the legislation has given drug addicts power to manipulate the healthcare system. The act holds physicians responsible for situations beyond their control. For example, if a doctor has a patient get a chest X-ray and treats the patient for an infection and the patient within 30 days goes to the hospital, the treating doctor, and the outpatient imaging facility will not be paid or will be expected to refund at least a portion of services paid for already. This is nonsense, yet part of the law. How does an outpatient facility even have a right or means to know if a person went to the hospital 29 days later? Fallout will likely be a lot more utilization of emergency services as outpatient physicians will have to be very selective in whom they treat and when to treat or not. Hence, a lot more patient information will be floating around cyberspace, meaning the law just made patient information less secure. Finally, under the ACA, even HIPAA gets more stringent and punitive. Now you do not even need a security breach of patient information to get in trouble, you only need to "appear to have an increased risk" of exposure of patient information. So now a non-event or narrowly avoided event is treated as if it actually happened and is punished even more severely than actual events. Small wonder there is a shortage of almost all healthcare providers in the United States.

The U.S. Supreme Court essentially considered the ACA unconstitutional as healthcare legislation, but acceptable as a taxation schematic.

So, not only does the Affordable Care Act not accomplish any of its publicized goals, it does not accomplish any of the huge potential savings while creating a more punitive and overregulated system.

Chapter 36
Legalized Marijuana

There is a big push to legalize marijuana use. Most marijuana discussions are highly emotional with little evidence. I can only tell you this: They call it dope for a reason. From a medical point of view, my experience in physical medicine and rehabilitation rotations showed me that many of the population seeking opioid prescriptions for pain tested positive for tetrahydrocannabinol (THC), a compound in marijuana. So, I guess my question is, "If marijuana is so great for pain control, why are you here asking for opioid medications for your pain?" It's a fair question, because so many people hype marijuana being the greatest pain reliever, yet I witnessed many pain patients self-medicating with marijuana still wanting prescription pain drugs. Perhaps the marijuana was effective, and they were just systematically lying to their doctor to get prescription drugs to sell on the street? If they were selling their prescription medications, then they were doing something morally wrong and illegal while under the influence of marijuana, which argues counter to statements that marijuana does not cloud judgment. Anyhow, the much-touted good effects and lack of bad effects regarding marijuana is counter to my witness. Anything going into your lungs other than fresh air is bad for your lungs.

Chapter 37
Medical Missions

I love doing medical missions work, because it is focused on just doing what you can to help people. The patient comes first. There is minimal documentation and facilities are limited, but the caring, compassion and appreciation of your efforts make it all worthwhile. Also, seeing what others consider "home" – cinderblock walls, a corrugated metal or plastic roof, rudimentary plumbing, unreliable electricity, and cardboard covering a dirt floor – makes me appreciative of the gifts God has given me and makes me appreciate the work of earlier generations of Americans who lived and died building the infrastructure so taken for granted these days. The conditions are less than 5-star, but hard work, love and a couple of meals a day makes it all worthwhile.

I remember at one site, when the electricity failed, within a few seconds there was a bunch of flashlights lit up and work continued. At the end of the evening, it was conversation, karaoke, occasionally basketball or soccer depending on your energy level. "Work hard and play hard" is how it was explained to me. Just as even God took a day of rest, after the mission work we take a Rest & Relaxation break somewhere for some hours or better part of a day to play or see the sights.

For me, doing missions work puts the humanity back into medicine, which over time has become dehumanized for doctor and patient.

Chapter 38
Was becoming a Doctor the Right Choice?

I don't know.

The End.

Epilogue

I remember a sign in a Catholic elementary school that stated: "What is right is not always popular, and what is popular is not always right." It was a very true statement then and remains so now, but I do hope that one day doing the right thing will also be popular.

I would also advise reading Fredrick Douglass' lecture *Self-Made Men* (1872). I mention this because honesty, integrity, hard work and success are now maligned characteristics in this country and advise you not to fall into such silly beliefs. The Self-Made Men lecture may also provide guidance to political leaders in creating a system encouraging creativity, innovation and productivity instead of killing such characteristics.

Follow your calling, because it is right for you and your humanity and self-worth, not because it may be popular, easy or financially rewarding. Success may not be easy, but fulfilling your vision of yourself brings its own rewards. We do not know the time of our final calling, but we can decide how we will live the present.